End Your Addiction Now

The Proven Nutritional Supplement Program That Can Set You Free

Charles Gant, MD
Greg Lewis, PhD

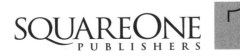

SQUAREONE
PUBLISHERS

Neither The Power Recovery Program nor any other program should be followed without first consulting a health care professional. If you have any special conditions requiring attention, you should consult with your health care professional regularly regarding possible modification of the program contained in this book.

Also, please note that the use of gendered pronouns in this book alternates by chapter. For example, when referencing a general person, the pronoun "he" will be used in one chapter and the pronoun "she" will be used in the next.

Cover Designer: Jeannie Tudor
Editor: Helene Ciaravino
Typesetter: Gary A. Rosenberg

Square One Publishers
Garden City Park, NY 11040 • (516)535-2010 • www.squareonepublishers.com

Library of Congress Cataloging-in-Publication Data

Gant, Charles.
    End your addiction now : the proven nutritional supplement program that can set you
free / by Charles Gant and Greg Lewis.
        p. cm.
    Includes index.
    ISBN 978-0-7570-0313-4
    1. Substance abuse--Nutritional aspects. I. Lewis, Greg. II. Title.
    RC564.29.G36 2010
    362.29--dc22
                                            2009022692

Printed in the United States of America.

10   9   8   7   6   5   4   3   2   1

Contents

Introduction

It's been only about a quarter of a century since we discovered that, contrary to what we'd thought for decades prior to that time, the brain actually sends signals from one neuron to another by means of chemical molecules, called neurotransmitters. That discovery has enabled us to put together the pieces of the puzzle of addiction in a way that we simply hadn't been able to do before we knew about these amazing chemical messengers.

Once we'd begun to understand how neurotransmitters work, we also began to understand how they control our moods, memory, thinking, and behavior. Each of our brain cells is a tiny but very powerful manufacturing plant that assembles these chemical molecules out of nutrients and passes them along to other neurons. When our brains have enough of the nutrients necessary to manufacture all of the neurotransmitters we need, we're able to feel relaxed and alert, focused and free of fear, happy and pain-free. In short, when our brains have the nutrients they need to create neurotransmitters in the necessary quantities, we're most fully alive, engaged, and productive.

When we're unable to produce neurotransmitters in the necessary quantities, our moods, intellectual capability, and behavior tend to deteriorate. We're often unable to focus, we tend to worry about things that we probably shouldn't be concerned with, we're not "up" and alert and happy, and we have difficulty coping with pain, whether the pain is physical or emotional. If neurotransmitter deficiencies persist over time, we're often led to use prescription drugs, alcohol, so-called "street drugs," and other substances, including nicotine, to substitute for our neurotransmitter shortages. These drugs are capable of temporarily alleviating the symptoms of neurotransmitter deficiencies, but continued use of these substances can, often quite quickly, result in addiction, a situation in which our brains adapt and begin to rely on these neurotransmitter substitutes to keep us going.

The problem is, of course, that drugs and alcohol are enormously harmful to us in so many ways. Rather than enabling us to function, they actually reduce our ability to perform without them. They alter our behavior and reduce our ability to experience the normal emotions of life. They ultimately cause depletions or diminished effects of the very neurotransmitters which they are meant to mimic or bolster.

Although the disciplines of medicine and psychiatry have understood neurotransmitters and how they work for quite some time, the primary use they've made of this information is to find ways to use prescription drugs to do the job that, prior to the biochemical revolution, could only be found through illicit drugs and legal substances such as alcohol and tobacco. They've given us Ritalin to control our kids' Attention Deficit Disorder (ADD), and Ritalin works in the brain in exactly the same way as cocaine. They've given us antidepressants such as Paxil and Prozac, which work in the brain to eventually shut down one of our most important neurotransmitters, a natural brain chemical that keeps us happy and relaxed. In short, they've pioneered "drug interventions." They've found ways to prescribe dozens, if not hundreds, of additional substances to which we can become very rapidly addicted. Indeed, the prescription drug problem in the United States is now much more severe and deadly than that of illicit drugs, and one of the main differences is that drug companies can now advertise their addictive drugs, while drug dealers can't. Young people now need go only as far as their parents' medicine cabinets to procure drugs that are often equally as powerful and addictive as those they can buy on the street.

Part One of this book introduces you to my Power Recovery Program, providing some important information to help you understand your brain's biochemistry and how disruptions in its natural biochemical processes can lead to substance abuse. You'll also learn about the three stages of the Power Recovery Program and how it can lead you back to addiction-free biochemical health.

Part Two of the book takes you through the first two stages of the Power Recovery Program, Quick-Start and Detoxification. These stages are designed to quickly reduce or eliminate your substance cravings and to enable you to get rid of the toxins that are most likely at the root of the biochemical imbalances that cause your substance cravings. Part Two also offers suggestions for maintaining the "healthier you" by making intelligent diet and nutrition decisions.

Part Three deals with what I call Long-Term Biochemical Rebalancing. It's designed to help you consolidate the positive changes you've brought about in the first two stages. It will also help those who've been using drugs and alcohol for long periods of time to diagnose and correct secondary conditions that may have resulted from the substance use.

Part Four will enable you to recognize many of the pitfalls of modern medical treatment, particularly the overuse of potentially addictive drugs in the treatment of psychological disorders and conditions such as Attention Deficit Disorder (ADD) and Attention Deficit/Hyperactivity Disorder (ADHD). It will provide you with the knowledge you need to resist the tendency of so many physicians to overmedicate their patients, especially children and young adults. Part Four also discusses a condition I call toxic overload, and explains how to treat it in safe and effective ways.

This book will help you understand how your brain works naturally and what you can do to restore its normal function and rid yourself or someone you love of the terrible burden of addiction. By following the step-by-step principles and practices outlined in this book, you can solve the puzzle of addiction and once again become a healthy, happy, drug-free person.

Part One

Introducing the Power Recovery Program

Part One of this book will give you a general overview of my Power Recovery Program. In Chapter 1, I'll provide several case histories of people who have developed substance problems and explain how they were able to use my program to overcome those difficulties and free themselves from their drug and alcohol use. You'll also find introductory material about the brain chemistry that underlies all addictions and how I've formulated a program of nutritional supplements to rebalance brain chemistry that's been disrupted by substance use. Chapter 1 also gives you an overview of the program's three stages, Quick-Start, Detoxification, and Long-Term Biochemical Rebalancing, and then answers many of the questions about the program that you may have.

Chapter 2 is designed to put the use of potentially addictive substances in an historical context, discussing how substance use evolved to the point at which technology enabled us to "supercharge" natural substances and make them much more addictive than they would normally be. I also talk about how I came to devote my career to helping people overcome their substance problems, and I provide additional information about how the Power Recovery Program can work in your life.

Chapter 3 goes into detail about how our bodies work at the cellular and molecular levels and how microscopic chemical reactions are the basis of every one of our daily activities. It also discusses our brain chemistry in greater detail, introducing the concept of neurotransmitters, which are brain chemicals that control how we think, feel, and behave. The chapter explains how nutritional imbalances can lead to imbalances in these important brain chemicals that make us susceptible to using drugs and alcohol.

Chapter 4 talks about why some people are more likely than others to become substance users, focusing on the four key risk factors for problem substance use. As part of this discussion, the chapter delves deeper into the subject of nutrition, explaining the importance of nutritional balance in our lives and introducing the idea that we can use nutritional supplements in order to achieve that balance.

This section of the book provides you with the background information you need to go ahead to Part Two, in which you will actually determine your own personal Power Recovery Program nutritional supplement plan. It's the foundation you need to begin your recovery.

1

A Revolution in the Treatment of Substance Use Problems

Over the past thirty years, I've helped thousands of patients recover successfully from nicotine, alcohol, stimulant, opiate, marijuana, and prescription drug addictions, as well as the addiction to carbohydrates and sugar, which I call "carboholism." In this book, I'll tell you more about the specifics of their treatments and show you the step-by-step program which enabled them to end their substance use, but let me begin this chapter by briefly presenting three case histories. These stories emphasize many of the difficulties my patients have experienced when trying to overcome their substance problems through conventional approaches. As is too often the case, those conventional approaches exacerbate substance problems . . . when they're not actually causing them. After I've reviewed these case histories, I'll dispel many of the myths about substance abuse that have held people back from successful recoveries. Then I'll give you an overview of the science behind my Power Recovery Program. Finally, I'll answer many of the questions I've heard from my patients over the years.

THREE PROFILES

Does the following story sound familiar to you?

Esther W. was embarrassed the first time she came into my office. "I just can't seem to quit smoking," she said. "I know there are so many people out there with worse problems than I have, I'm almost ashamed to tell you about mine." Esther had started smoking when she was a junior in high school, to be "one of the crowd," as she put it. That was fifteen years ago. She knew about the dangers: "I can read the warnings on the packs. I just can't make myself take them seriously," she said.

It had gotten to the point where she worried that she was harming the health of the other members of her family, particularly her two small children. She also confessed that she felt as if her husband, who had quit smoking the year before, no longer found her as attractive as he once had, and that he'd hinted that her smoking was the primary reason. Esther had tried hypnosis, acupuncture, and a stop-smoking program sponsored by the American Lung Association. I could feel her frustration as she said, "I guess the straw that broke the camel's back for me was when our family doctor prescribed a nicotine patch for me. Isn't nicotine what I'm addicted to? How am I supposed to quit using an addictive substance when all my doctor does is give me a prescription for the same stuff?"

Or perhaps you've experienced something like this:

Michael M. was 11 years old when his parents first brought him to see me. Within a few minutes of meeting him, I realized Michael was above average in intelligence. He got As and Bs in all of his subjects, but when I asked him about his classes he replied, "Bo-oring."

Michael had been identified as a boy with potential behavioral problems by his third and fourth grade teachers. He had gone to a child psychologist once a week for three months in the Spring semester of fourth grade, but his unacceptable behavior didn't change. Early in his second semester in fifth grade, Michael's parents were called to a meeting with his teacher and the school psychologist. The teacher reported that Michael's classroom behavior had become "too disruptive." In Michael's teacher's words, "He's constantly fidgeting, and he rarely pays attention in class. He just doesn't seem to have a normal attention span." Both the teacher and the school psychologist recommended that Michael's parents consider "putting him on Ritalin."

His parents took Michael to see their pediatrician. After a ten-minute consultation, the pediatrician told them that Michael was suffering from Attention Deficit Hyperactivity Disorder (ADHD) and gave them a prescription for Ritalin for Michael. Michael's classroom behavior got "better," meaning he didn't fidget as much, and his behavior was deemed less disruptive by his teacher. His grades improved marginally, but Michael still thought school was not very interesting. Every day, by the time his afternoon dose of Ritalin had worn off early in the evening, Michael became irritable and unable to concentrate or sit still. His parents decided to live with this behavior, considering they were no longer hearing complaints from school.

When school let out for the summer, and his parents tried to taper his Ritalin usage, Michael began to show hostility towards those around him, and again became easily irritated and unable to concentrate. The family doctor advised his parents to keep him on the drug. They even saw a column in the local newspaper that recommended keeping kids on Ritalin during summer vacation. It was Michael who finally opened their eyes. "I don't want to take this stuff," he said. "I can't help it if I'm active. It's just me. I don't want to be a Ritalin geek, but I don't like it when I don't take it. I feel horrible."

Or maybe you've encountered a situation like this one:

Jane L. is a 28-year-old woman who started her own public relations business and was working very hard to build it up. "It's just me and a secretary right now, but it's really beginning to grow," she told me proudly. The pride turned to sadness when she began to discuss her drinking problem. She and her husband had separated, then divorced, a little over two years ago. To cope with the stress of her divorce and the uncertainty of starting her own business, she began to have a glass or two of wine every night. She told me it helped her relax. Within a few months, she was drinking a bottle of wine every evening. She was exhausted every day because she was trying to recover from a hangover while she conducted her business. She started looking forward to weekends, when she could "really unwind." Translation: Drink even more heavily.

Jane began going to a therapist to get help coping with the depression she hadn't really been able to break out of since her divorce. After several months of consultations proved largely ineffective, her therapist recommended Prozac, which Jane's physician willingly prescribed. When I first met her, Jane had been taking the drug for five months, during which time she also continued to drink to excess. When the subject of her drinking came up, the therapist at first told her, "You're not psychologically ready to quit using prescription drugs or alcohol." As her drinking worsened, the therapist began to tell her, "You don't want to quit badly enough," and "Once you've worked through your psychological problems, you'll have a much better chance of stopping your drinking."

ANALYZING THE MESSAGE OF CONVENTIONAL TREATMENT STRATEGIES

Let me start by pointing out several things about these people that virtually all of my patients have in common. First, they are all good people who began to use addictive substances for what seemed like justifiable reasons and who found that their substance use was causing problems. The message here is that you don't have to be an "addict" to have a problem with addictive substances.

Second, they had all received counseling and/or treatment from traditional sources, such as psychotherapists, school psychologists, and family physicians. Third, their treatment strategies had them using potentially addictive mood-altering substances, including nicotine, Ritalin, and Prozac. In each case, the substances were supposed to help them overcome their primary problems. Finally, they were unable to find solutions to their problems through traditional methods.

These brief case histories highlight two important tendencies. The first is the consistent failure of traditional approaches in treating substance use problems. The second is the growing tendency among physicians to put their patients *at risk* by prescribing potentially addictive mood-altering substances, substances which at best *temporarily* mask behavioral and substance use problems. At worst, the patients whom these prescription drugs are supposed to help actually become addicted to the prescription drugs themselves. These trends have led many people to question whether traditional approaches really work. The answer is not just a simple "yes" or "no."

There's no doubt that traditional drug and alcohol treatment strategies used by most physicians and in most drug and alcohol rehabilitation facilities have enjoyed *some* success. On average, around 25 percent of the people who use these traditional methods do recover. But there's a catch: Research data suggests that approximately 20 percent of all substance abusers recover *with no treatment at all*. In any case, if you have a substance problem, your chance of recovery through traditional methods is about one in four, and I think those are lousy odds. Whether it's your therapist, your MD, or your Alcoholics Anonymous (AA) sponsor, he is in effect saying to you, "Do it my way. I'll help you recover." What they're not saying is that you may recover if you're the lucky one in four patients. I think you deserve better.

I've dedicated my medical career to treating compulsive substance users, from smokers to alcoholic and drug-dependent people to bulimic and anorexic "carboholics." I became frustrated very early by the obvious inadequacies of traditional methods used by most of the addictions, medical, and psychiatric treatment community, and this frustration led me to begin closely following the exciting new scientific research in the field of biochemistry. It is this research—virtually ignored by most healthcare professionals—that has become the basis for my revolutionary new substance abuse treatment strategy, the *Power Recovery Program*. This program takes full advantage of what the research has taught us, and it has consistently achieved outstanding recovery rates.

The proof of this is in the results. While I was Medical Director of the Tully Hill Hospital, a fifty-six-bed, JCAH-approved (Joint Commission for the Accreditation of Hospitals) drug and alcohol detoxification and rehabilitation facility near Syracuse, New York, I developed a treatment program that incorporated totally natural nutritional supplements (including nutrients such as amino acids, vitamins, and minerals) into the overall treatment plans for thousands of patients. This nutritional supplementation protocol was based on the revolutionary new discoveries in biochemistry to which I've referred. According to a clinical outcome study conducted by New Standards, Inc., an independent research group which assesses drug and alcohol recovery results, more than 80 percent of the patients who followed through with the nutritional protocols I implemented remained alcohol- and drug-free a full year after completing their treatment. That's over three times better than the national average when conventional methods are used. These results suggest that with the Power Recovery Program, the odds are as high as five to one that you will be able to successfully overcome your substance use problem.

EXPLODING SOME MYTHS ABOUT SUBSTANCE USE

The primary reason my patients have been able to achieve such dramatic results using the Power Recovery Program is that I've developed a plan that avoids what I call "the four myths about compulsive substance use." Let me dispel these myths right now:

Myth 1: Compulsive substance use is a sign of lack of will power, or of an underlying moral or spiritual problem.

Myth 2: Drugs and alcohol are the causes of substance abuse.

Myth 3: Chronic substance users are "victims" of a disease which can be treated as we treat other diseases: with prescription drugs.

Myth 4: Once you've successfully stopped using drugs or alcohol, you have to engage in a constant struggle not to relapse.

None of these myths is true, but most physicians and counselors specializing in alcohol and drug rehabilitation will tell you that they are. They've become the cornerstone beliefs of almost all traditional approaches. In fact they're rationalizations which are often used as excuses for the ineffectiveness of the addiction treatment strategies of the past fifty years or so. Let me put it another way: If you were a doctor and able to cure only about 25 percent of the patients you treated, of course you'd think that the condition you were treating was a very difficult one. And if you started with the idea that the condition you were treating resulted from a moral weakness in your patients, your approach to the condition would reflect that idea. It's called a self-fulfilling prophecy. If you subscribed wholeheartedly, as most doctors do, to the idea that all diseases were caused by outside agents such as germs, and that by taking medications to control these agents you could control disease, it would be a small jump to call substance problems "diseases" caused by nicotine, alcohol, and other drugs, and to attempt to treat them with prescription drugs, as you treated other diseases.

Clearly, traditional approaches are producing unacceptable recovery rates in large part because they're based on incorrect assumptions about the nature of substance problems. I've been able to avoid these pitfalls with the Power Recovery Program because I've translated recent biochemical research into a revolutionary approach which treats substance problems where they really happen: at the cellular and molecular levels.

Let me give you some background. Every one of the tens of trillions of cells in our bodies functions according to an ancient and complex set of biochemical laws that have been evolving for billions of years. Most of these cells have become highly specialized, performing one or a small number of very specific tasks. Within each individual cell in our bodies, millions of chemical reactions occur every second. Each of the requires a specific combination of nutrients, in precisely the right in order to take place. If we're not getting the nutrients we need, w not be supplying our cells with the raw materials they need to carry it their complex chemistry. This can result in a condition of biochemical imbalance, and it can cause our physical and mental health to deteriorate if left uncorrected.

Imbalances are particularly important in the biochemistry of brain cells, or neurons. Neurons produce chemical substances called *neurotransmitters*. These substances are the brain's messengers, and by exchanging neurotransmitters among themselves, neurons control virtually every aspect of our lives. Several key neurotransmitters, which I'll discuss in more detail in this and following chapters, affect our moods and behavior dramatically. When the brain is unable to produce them in adequate supply due to lack of adequate nutrition, or when toxins (including environmental toxins, nicotine, alcohol, and other drugs) compromise their normal activity, or when illness or stress depletes them, we may feel restless, depressed, angry, or agitated, or be unable to focus or concentrate. So common are these feelings among people who abuse drugs and alcohol that, if you have a substance problem, you probably recognize them in yourself. Perhaps you use drugs or alcohol to help overcome them.

DRUGS AND ALCOHOL: SHORT-CIRCUITING BRAIN CHEMISTRY

Potentially addictive substances, including nicotine, alcohol, cocaine, heroin, marijuana, Prozac, and Valium, to name only a few, function by short-circuiting brain chemistry. Their chemical structures are such that they literally substitute for the neurotransmitters the brain may be unable to produce in adequate amounts. That is, they make us temporarily feel better and change our behavior by "fooling" the brain into thinking it is producing enough of certain neurotransmitters.

Let me give you an example of how this process works. The neurotransmitter dopamine has a powerful effect on the way we feel and behave. When brain cells are producing and utilizing this neurotransmitter in adequate amounts, we feel focused and alert. Dopamine also enables us to get the fullest enjoyment from pleasurable experiences.

Under normal circumstances, our brain cells use nutrients to produce billions of molecules of dopamine every second. This assembly takes place according to a formula that does not vary. If there is a shortage of even one of the necessary nutrients, dopamine cannot be produced in adequate amounts, potentially causing us to have difficulty concentrating, putting us in a bad mood, and inhibiting our ability to enjoy life's everyday activities. A number of drugs, cocaine and Ritalin in particular, act as substitutes for dopamine, temporarily making us feel the way we would feel if our brains were producing dopamine in adequate amounts.

In short, based on my medical practice and the scientific research of the past twenty-five years, I have come to understand that substance problems are primarily the result of biochemical imbalances which disrupt the normal workings of brain cells.

Most addictions treatment professionals believe incorrectly that substance use problems are caused only by emotional and psychological factors, or by the substances themselves. In fact, scientific research has shown that substance cravings, mood swings, sleep problems, symptoms of mental disorders, and dysfunctional behaviors are largely driven by biochemical imbalances that disrupt the production of neurotransmitters. The imbalances result when our brains are unable to get the nutrients they need to produce adequate amounts of neurotransmitters, or when toxins interfere with normal brain metabolism and neurotransmitter function. Through the Power Recovery Program, these imbalances can be corrected and normal neurotransmitter production restored by making sure our brains are supplied with the natural nutrients they need and by removing toxins which have accumulated in the brain. The key component of the Program is taking specific nutritional supplements which provide the brain with the raw materials it needs to rebalance its biochemistry. In other words, the most critical component in recovering from compulsive substance use is rebalancing brain chemistry. Many studies, which are documented in the Bibliography section of this book, provide conclusive evidence that this is true, and my experience in successfully treating thousands of patients for the past two decades confirms it.

As you can imagine, in the light of this new knowledge about the biochemistry of addictions, we've had to significantly change what we mean by the word "recovery." The recovery process is frequently described as the restoration of body, mind, and spirit. The problem is that many programs have focused only on the latter two and have ignored the "body" component of recovery. Addictions are physical substances causing physical changes to a physical organ, the brain. So how do we conventionally treat them? With group therapy and spiritual counseling. Doesn't make sense, does it?

Recovery does not consist simply of a psychological or spiritual transformation, as most traditional treatment programs would define it. The foundation of successful recovery is treating the "body" component of addiction through the re-establishment of normal brain chemistry. That chemistry may have become disrupted through the prolonged use of one or more toxic substances, including alcohol, drugs, and cigarettes; by toxins in the environment; by physical or emotional stress; by nutritional deficiencies; or because of a genetic predisposition. The key to unlocking the door to recovery is getting your brain chemistry back to normal, and when that has been accomplished, the recovery of mind and spirit can much more readily take place. The Power Recovery Program shows you how to take the critical first step in eliminating the need for drugs and alcohol in your life by using only natural nutrients to rebalance your biochemistry.

HOW CAN THE POWER RECOVERY PROGRAM HELP ME?

The Power Recovery Program has one purpose: To help you, as a recovering substance user, improve your outcome, regardless of what else you do. By "improve your outcome," I mean dramatically increase the odds that you'll be able to successfully recover from your substance problem. You'll notice that I haven't said that you need to abandon any treatment strategy you're using now. If you're following a traditional recovery strategy, you've got about a one-in-four chance of success. If you combine that strategy with the Power Recovery Program, the evidence suggests that you'll increase your chances of recovery to five out of six. Even if you're not currently following a recovery plan, my clinical experience in prescribing the Power Recovery Program to thousands of patients strongly suggests that you'll dramatically improve your chances for a complete recovery. The Program is unique because you can use it as a standalone strategy, or you can combine it with any other program you're currently following.

The three patients whose case histories I outlined at the beginning of this chapter will give you a good idea of the different ways the Power

Recovery Program can work. Both Jane and Esther decided to discontinue the programs they were following. After our first appointment, Esther immediately stopped using her nicotine patch. Within twenty-four hours of beginning the Power Recovery Program, her cravings for cigarettes had completely disappeared. "It took me about two months to become a nonsmoker," she said, "but it only took one day to quit cigarettes." She went on to explain what she meant by "becoming a nonsmoker": "I had to get over all the little habits associated with smoking, like reaching for a cigarette in my purse, or thinking I needed a cigarette after dinner. I didn't crave cigarettes at all. But I had to get over going through the motions of smoking, and that was possible because I'd gotten over my moodiness and I didn't have the urge to smoke."

Michael's parents' first reaction when they realized their son had a substance problem was one of anger. They felt as if they had been coerced into putting their son on Ritalin without having been given adequate background information. They were unaware, for instance, that Ritalin is a controlled substance, classified, along with morphine and methamphetamine, as one of the most addictive substances known. In fact, Ritalin works to disrupt brain chemistry in exactly the same way cocaine does. Fortunately, Michael's experience has a very positive resolution. The results of a series of diagnostic tests I prescribed for him showed the real roots of Michael's behavior problems: he had elevated lead levels (heavy metal poisoning), as well as digestive problems that prevented him from absorbing certain nutrients in his food.

His father's response was, "I may not be a doctor, but this simply makes perfect medical sense to me. Why didn't our family doctor discover these things?" Unfortunately, the answer is that he didn't look for them. Michael's doctor went for what I call "the ten-minute solution." He did a cursory examination, then followed what has become the "accepted standard of care" among physicians—he prescribed Ritalin. It's modern medicine's equivalent of the Old West gunslinger's creed: "Prescribe first, ask questions later." Within two weeks of beginning the regimen of nutritional supplements designed to detoxify his body and restore his impaired digestive function, Michael no longer needed Ritalin, and his behavior had improved remarkably. His mother's comment sums the situation up: "He's actually behaving better now than he did when he was taking Ritalin."

Jane was able to stop drinking almost immediately and taper her Prozac dosage down to nothing within two weeks after she began taking the Power Recovery Program nutrients. Within three weeks, her attitude had brightened significantly. "You know," she said, "My situation hasn't changed that much, but I really feel like I can cope with it now. For the first time in two years, I'm in touch with my feelings and not masking them with alcohol or prescription drugs." Jane began to see another therapist who understood the benefits of the Power Recovery Program and worked with Jane to help her deal with her true feelings.

I've talked about the low success rates of traditional addictions treatment programs, and now we're in a position to understand why those success rates are low. As I've said, simply put, none of the traditional strategies takes into account the *biochemical basis* of substance abuse. While no one denies that there are emotional and psychological components to many, if not most, substance problems, the fact remains that if you ignore the biochemical component of substance use, you can expend tremendous resources on psychological and emotional support and still not get to the primary causes of the substance problem.

WHAT'S THE SCIENTIFIC BASIS OF THE POWER RECOVERY PROGRAM?

The laws of biochemistry are absolute and unchanging, and we live according to them, whether we know it or not. By following my Power Recovery Program, you'll be getting yourself back in synch with what I refer to as "your billion-year-old biochemistry."

Indeed, one important aspect of life is the biochemical aspect; it can be said that life is essentially a chemical process. Our biochemistry has evolved over billions of years to become an extraordinarily complex set of chemical interactions. As our knowledge of this biochemistry increases, we're learning how to correct disruptions to it and restore its normal functions without the use of toxic substances, including carbohydrates, alcohol, and "recreational" and prescription drugs. In the process, we're beginning to understand that biochemistry is the key to health and that restoring normal biochemical functions is the key to eliminating diseases and disease-like conditions. We're also learning that the best way to restore our physical and mental health is by providing our bodies and brains with the natural nutrients they need. As we've seen, the biochemical basis of addictions rests in nutritional deficiencies which prevent our brains from functioning normally.

THE STAGES OF THE POWER RECOVERY PROGRAM

The Power Recovery Program has three stages:

The first stage of the Power Recovery Program, called Quick-Start, reduces or eliminates your drug and alcohol cravings within twenty-four to seventy-two hours. It enables you, through simple questionnaires, to identify specific nutrient deficiencies which are the true causes of your substance cravings and other symptoms. It then provides you with a program of nutritional supplements which will raise the levels of those nutrients in your body and quickly enable your brain to resume producing neurotransmitters more normally. The most dramatic effect of the Quick-Start stage is that your drug and/or alcohol cravings can be significantly reduced or even eliminated very quickly, usually in one to three days, enabling you to concentrate on the other aspects of your recovery plan. Even if you're in recovery and have not abused drugs or alcohol for years, you may still have biochemical imbalances and symptoms which Quick-Start can help you overcome.

The Detoxification stage of the Power Recovery Program works to rid your body of many common types of toxins, not just those resulting from drug use. Toxic substances have accumulated in your body as a result of substance abuse, but you may also have high levels of toxins in your body as a result of environmental pollution, dental fillings, and pesticides and chemical additives in the food you eat. In fact, high levels of toxins from these and other sources often *cause* biochemical imbalances in the first place, by damaging our digestive tracts or by interfering with our cellular biochemistry. In addition, many addicts and drug users have poor eating habits; their diets are often unbalanced, and they tend to eat excessive quantities of sugar and other refined carbohydrates. Over time this can cause disruptions in brain chemistry that lead to or exacerbate drug cravings. In stage two you will begin a second regimen of nutritional supplements that will help you cleanse your system of toxins.

The third stage of the Power Recovery Program is titled Long-Term Biochemical Rebalancing. It enables you to deal not just with the group of nutrient deficiencies which is disrupting your brain chemistry, but also with other *secondary* nutritional imbalances. If these latter imbalances are left uncorrected, they might eventually result in a return of your substance cravings.

As you progress with the Power Recovery Program, you'll move through each of these three stages, and at each one you will find yourself feeling more focused and alert. As you provide your body with the nutrients it needs, you will experience the benefits of letting your natural biochemical processes take care of the healing that is the very core of successful recovery.

ANSWERING SOME QUESTIONS ABOUT THE POWER RECOVERY PROGRAM

If you're like most people, when you hear that there's an addiction recovery program that will reduce substance cravings, detoxify your body, and help heal the biochemical damage done by drug and alcohol abuse—and do it all using only natural nutritional supplements—you're probably somewhat skeptical. And you've probably got a lot of questions. I've compiled the questions, along with their answers, that I'm asked most frequently by my patients.

Q. How do I know your program is going to work? Are there any studies that document the success of this approach?

A. Tens of thousands of my patients and others have used the Power Recovery Program to support successful recoveries from their alcohol and substance problems. The Bibliography section at the end of this book includes an extensive list of books and articles published in peer-reviewed journals which show that nutritional supplementation not only helps in recovery but may be the most important part of any recovery plan. In fact, studies suggest that the biochemical imbalances which nutritional supplements can correct are, in themselves, the direct causes of addiction.

Q. Why hasn't anyone told me about using nutrients to help me overcome my substance problem? Should I tell my doctor or my counselor or my AA sponsor I'm taking these nutrients? Should I continue other treatment programs along with the Power Recovery Program?

A. While in medical school, your doctor, if his experience was like mine, had less than one hour of training on the subject of nutrition. Physicians are taught to give highest priority to diagnosing and treating acute and life-threatening medical problems. Chronic medical problems, especially those resulting from nutritional and biochemical imbalances and exposure to toxins, are, by necessity, given lower priority. Unless your doctor has done a great deal of independent study on the subject of nutrition since then, he is really not qualified to comment on the nutritional basis of addictions. Couple that with the medical profession's overwhelming bias toward using prescription drugs—which is the preferred and appropriate treatment strategy for acute medical problems—and you'll understand why you've not heard about treating addictions using nutritional supplements. In fact, the damage done by prescription drug abuse now exceeds that of alcohol, smoking, and illegal drug use.

Like your physician, most people in substance support groups like Alcoholics Anonymous have had no training in nutrition. It's not their fault that they're unable to inform you about this approach to treating addictions. My own case is a good example. Since I received almost no education about nutrition in medical school, I had to do a tremendous amount of independent research to learn about human biochemistry and the ways nutrition affects it. That research has led me to develop the Power Recovery Program.

I would encourage you to discuss my Power Recovery Program with your doctor or counselor. I'd especially recommend that you make them aware of the books and articles referenced in the Bibliography, so that they can appreciate the scientific basis of my approach. I also encourage you to continue with any spiritual or psychological programs you're currently pursuing, if you feel they're aiding your recovery. These programs, such as Alcoholics Anonymous, will give you emotional support while my Power Recovery Program will improve the biochemical foundation on which your recovery is based.

Q. My doctor told me I have a genetic predisposition for alcoholism. Can the Power Recovery Program still help me?

A. The Power Recovery Program is the *only* kind of recovery program which directly addresses genetic predispositions for chemical dependencies. If you've been told that you have a genetic predisposition for alcoholism or any other chemical dependence, this simply means that you are more genetically vulnerable to specific nutritional deficiencies and that your reactions when you're exposed to certain toxins are more severe than those of most other people. Those who are genetically vulnerable to these conditions must pay closer attention to their nutritional requirements and minimize exposure to toxins such as alcohol and drugs and junk food. Where genetic vulnerability is extreme, people must avoid exposure to drugs and alcohol completely.

Q. I've been a smoker and a heavy drinker for twenty-five years. Is it too late to start taking these nutrients?

A. It's not too late at all. In fact, it's more important than ever. As we age, our ability to ward off injury from toxins in the environment is lessened, and our nutritional requirements increase. These conditions are made worse by nicotine, alcohol, and drug use. Even in long-term substance users, though, biochemical imbalances are correctable by using the nutrients in the Power Recovery Program. Your incredibly resilient biochemistry is designed to heal itself when it is properly nourished and detoxified.

Q. I heard that the Food and Drug Administration had banned some amino acids. Are these nutrients safe?

A. Only one amino acid, tryptophan, has ever been banned, and it was banned, not because of any problem with the amino acid itself, but because of contaminants in one batch of tryptophan from a particular manufacturer. Tryptophan is now available again over the counter. As you know, we eat all the amino acids, including tryptophan, every day as part of our regular diet. Amino acids are in virtually all the foods we consume, and are absolutely necessary nutrients to support life. Amino acids, along with the other nutrients in my Power Recovery Program, are naturally occurring substances which are not only harmless but necessary for good health.

Q. Can I do your program at home, or will I need to check into a hospital?

A. The Power Recovery Program can be done at home or in the hospital. If you are at risk for severe withdrawal symptoms from certain substances, especially alcohol and drugs such as Xanax, Klonopin, Ativan, Valium, and Librium, to mention several, you should seek professional help, which might include hospitalization. If you're not at risk for severe withdrawal, you can safely do the Power Recovery Program at home. (I'll discuss this further in Chapter 6.) Whatever your choice, the Power Recovery Program will improve your outcome.

Q. I smoke cigarettes because they help me concentrate. I'm afraid if I stop smoking I won't be able to get my work done.

A. Nicotine, the addictive substance in cigarettes, artificially stimulates receptors for several different neurotransmitters. If you smoke cigarettes, your brain overcompensates for the presence of nicotine by producing less of these neurotransmitters, relying on nicotine to do the job the neurotransmitters are designed to do. The Power Recovery Program resupplies your brain with the nutrients needed to jump-start the production of these neurotransmitters. This means that, instead of relying on cigarettes to help you concentrate, your brain will be able to produce the neurotransmitters that enable you to focus naturally, without nicotine. Not only do most people experience no reduction in their ability to concentrate when they stop using cigarettes with the Power Recovery Program, but also they find that their ability to concentrate is improved, even without cigarettes.

Q. How will the nutrients make me feel? Will they make me tired? Give me more energy?

A. It's important to understand that nutrients themselves don't make you *feel* a certain way. What they do is enable your brain and body chemistry to begin working properly so that you actually experience your own feelings and not feelings that are temporarily and artificially induced by the presence of toxins, such as nicotine, alcohol, and drugs, in your brain, or by the absence of neurotransmitters due to nutritional deficiencies. Our biochemistry is designed to keep us alert, focused, and full of energy. When we get enough of the proper nutrients, our brains and bodies will take care of the rest, making us feel the way nature intended.

Q. How will I know the nutrients are working? Are there tests I should have to determine whether they're working?

A. First, if followed correctly, there is almost no way that the Power Recovery Program nutrients won't work, unless your body and brain are so highly toxic that you're unable to absorb and utilize them properly. (This is dealt with in Chapters 6 and 17.) Most of the nutrients you'll be taking are almost certainly missing or in short supply in your diet. They're especially important in supporting recovery. Everyone responds somewhat differently to the nutrients. You may find that they improve your mood and frame of mind dramatically, or the effects on you may be more subtle. I've known many cases where the first people to notice the positive differences in the mood and behavior of people using the Power Recovery Program were family and friends. Whether the differences in how you feel are subtle or startling, stay with the Power Recovery Program. You can only benefit by it.

There are a number of tests which can help you pinpoint your nutritional deficiencies with great accuracy. These tests are discussed in Part Three, which deals with long-term biochemical rebalancing.

Q. Can I overdose on any of the Power Recovery Program nutrients or develop a dependence on them? What happens when I quit taking them?

A. It's virtually impossible to overdose on the Power Recover Program nutrients in the quantities recommended. Since they are nutrients, your body has developed natural ways of getting rid of them if they are present in excessive amounts. As you increase the amount of nutrients you take in, your body's reserve levels of those nutrients increase so they're available when needed.

These increased levels of nutrients mean that your body can use them when necessary, in times of physical or emotional stress, for instance. Over time, you will be able to reduce the amounts of nutritional supplements you take and still realize the benefits of healthy brain chemistry.

Alcohol and drugs are mind-altering toxins which actually deplete the levels of nutrients in your body, which causes you to crave more of them to compensate for decreased nutrient levels. That's why you can become dependent on drugs, and why you can't develop the same kind of dependence on nutrients. If you stop taking the nutritional supplements, your body will go on extracting nutrients from the foods you eat and benefiting from the nutrients that have built up as a result of taking supplements. Depending on your diet, toxin exposure, stress levels, and genetics, you may eventually deplete your nutrient stores again, if you've stopped taking nutritional supplements. Just resume your Power Recovery Program supplements to modify substance cravings, mood swings, sleep problems, or other symptoms that may have reoccurred.

Q. What if I'm allergic to some of the nutrients? Are there any foods I should avoid when I'm taking the nutrients?

A. The nutrients I recommend for the Power Recovery Program are completely natural and non-allergenic. It is extremely unusual for anyone to be allergic to these nutrients, because they are freer of allergy-causing substances than almost any other food in your regular diet. There are foods that you should avoid, not just while you're doing the Power Recovery Program, but at all times. Primary among these are "junk foods," meaning highly processed foods that are high in sugar and empty carbohydrates and chemical additives and preservatives. (If you do continue eating junk foods and abusing alcohol and drugs, you'll need nutritional supplements more than ever.)

I'm confident that the answers to these questions will address many of the concerns you might have had about the Power Recovery Program. As you proceed with the book, you'll find further information that will expand on the answers I've given here and help you to better understand the issues they raise. This will give you the confidence you need to go ahead with your own successful recovery.

CONCLUSION

In this chapter, I've highlighted some of the reasons that so many people have difficulty overcoming their substance problems. Conventional medicine is certainly one of the culprits in this. From its perverse insistence on using potentially addictive substances in treating substance abuse problems to its unwillingness to recognize that its methods are not producing acceptable results, conventional medicine has in too many cases made the "solution" worse than the original problem.

I've also, though, begun to focus on the only proven way to reduce substance cravings and eliminate your need to use potentially addictive substances. The Power Recovery Program, with its aim of rebalancing brain chemistry using only natural means, now provides people looking for solutions to their substance problems with a safe, proven alternative method that promises to return them to good health and restore the balance in their lives that substance abuse has upset.

2

How Has Substance Use Been Treated Historically?

I've used the term "substance" several times in Chapter 1. Even though most people have a fairly good idea of what is meant by the word, in this chapter I want to give you a definition of the term "substance" that will help you understand why I place so much emphasis in my Power Recovery Program on rebalancing brain chemistry. I also want to briefly trace the use of substances throughout history so that you'll get an idea of just how important they have been in the lives of our ancestors and how they've become such an important aspect of our lives today.

THE TERM "SUBSTANCE"

When I use the word "substance," I'm referring specifically to a *psychotropic* substance. A *psychotropic substance* is one which *interacts directly with brain cells* to influence moods, thoughts, and behavior. All psychotropic substances are potentially addictive.

The list of concentrated, potentially addictive psychotropic substances with which I'll be dealing in this book is quite long. It includes the following:

• Nicotine, primarily in the form of cigarettes.

• Alcohol.

• Stimulants, including cocaine, amphetamines, and many prescription drugs, such as Ritalin.

• Prescription mood-altering drugs, especially antidepressant and anti-anxiety drugs such as Prozac, Paxil, and Valium, among others.

• Opiates, including heroin and prescription painkillers such as morphine and Demerol.

• Psychedelics, including marijuana, mescaline, and LSD.

• Carbohydrates, especially sugar but also including so-called "complex carbohydrates."

Regarding the last entry, although carbohydrates are not psychotropic substances, they are highly addictive and can trigger disruptions in normal brain chemistry. In addition, with our average consumption rate of sugar now greater than 100 pounds per person per year, carbohydrates are one of the most abused substances in America today.

I'm concerned with these major categories of psychotropic substances because, in the concentrated forms in which they're available today, they're all capable of triggering compulsive use. With prolonged use, they're also capable of causing long-term changes in brain function as well as brain injury.

I first realized the potentially devastating effects of substance abuse in the mid-1970s, shortly after I completed medical school. As part of a scholarship agreement, I was employed by the United States Public Health Service to provide medical services to underserved populations in the southwestern United States. I expected to treat routine medical conditions, but I quickly discovered that most of the problems with which my patients came to me were directly connected with drug and alcohol abuse. These problems ranged from malnutrition to psychological disorders—including depression, bipolar illness, and schizophrenia—to degenerative medical conditions resulting from substance abuse. Like most students of the '70s, I was aware of "recreational" drug and alcohol use on college campuses, but nothing I had seen could have prepared me for what I encountered in my first professional appointment as an MD.

This experience proved to be my awakening to two things. The first was the devastating effects of alcohol and drug abuse. I began to recognize that excessive alcohol consumption, in particular, was the primary condition underlying many of the most prevalent medical and psychiatric disorders among the people I was treating, and that finding a way to help my patients overcome their substance problems would be the key to eliminating a significant number of their general health problems.

The second realization was that my conventional medical training had left me totally unprepared to treat medical and psychiatric problems caused by substance abuse. I began to understand that, while I had been trained to treat such disorders by giving patients prescription drugs (which, I would later discover, actually added to their problems), I had no knowledge of how to treat them by helping them *stop* using the alcohol and drugs which were the underlying causes of their medical problems.

Like all American physicians, I had been trained to prescribe, prescribe, prescribe. The clinic cabinets were stocked with powerful prescription psychotropic drugs, from Valium to Thorazine, and since I was also the resident pharmacist, I did what I'd been taught to do. I prescribed. The result was that I made no positive impact whatsoever on the root causes of most of the medical problems my patients were experiencing. To this day I regret the fact that I wasn't able to help, and I'm certain that this is one of the factors that led me to devote my career to helping people overcome substance problems.

NATURE, SUBSTANCES, AND SURVIVAL

While substance *abuse* almost always has some negative consequences, substance *use* is not necessarily a negative or damaging thing. In fact, the ancestors of the very people for whom I was providing medical services in the mid-1970s had a long history of using psychotropic substances, including peyote and magic mushrooms, to induce visions in their religious rituals. And tobacco has been and continues to be revered as a sacred substance by many Native American people, who regularly use it without abuse. In fact, psychotropic substances had been a part of nature long before the appearance of humans on our planet.

Psychotropic substances no doubt originated as survival mechanisms for certain plants. One of the more effective of these survival methods has proven to be appetite suppression. Tobacco, coca, poppy, and coffee plants, to name just a few with which most people are familiar, all contain substances which interact with and alter the biochemistry of the nervous systems of the creatures which consume their leaves, seeds, or flowers. These substances—nicotine, cocaine, morphine, and caffeine respectively—all have the effect of, among other things, very quickly suppressing the appetites of those who consume them. When an insect begins to eat the leaves of a tobacco plant, for example, it ingests nicotine, which alters the chemistry of its nervous system. The insect's perception of its condition changes rapidly from "I feel uncomfortable and hungry" to "I'm satisfied," even if it has just begun eating. By producing a chemical that makes the insect stop eating its leaves, the plant is protected from being destroyed before it has a chance to mature and reproduce.

There's an interesting sidelight to this story. As anyone will tell you who has tried to quit smoking, only to find that he or she gains weight, nicotine is an appetite suppressant in humans as well. Nicotine alters chemicals in the human nervous system to make smokers less hungry, *the exact same chemicals as those in many insects' nervous systems.* As you read through this book, you'll find numerous examples—like the one I've just given—of how, when nature finds a biochemical process that is successful, it is used over and over again for the same purpose in other creatures.

As I've said, psychotropic substances occur throughout nature, and the controlled use of psychotropic substances has been and continues to be a part of the lives of the people of virtually every society and culture on earth. Just as many indigenous North American peoples use tobacco and psychedelic substances in religious rituals, indigenous people of the Andes Mountains regularly chew the leaves of coca plants—from which cocaine is derived—to help combat fatigue and hunger. The relatively small doses of cocaine they ingest in this way are strong enough to provide benefits, and use of the substance is limited to controlled situations.

In addition to psychotropic substances occurring in nature, fermented beverages have been part of human culture for more than 8,000 years. From early beers—in which grains mixed with water were accidentally fermented by yeast in the air that settled on the mixture—to modern beers brewed in sterile stainless steel vats, this alcoholic drink has provided sustenance and relief to the people of virtually every culture in history. And for the past 6,500 years, wine has been part of the cuisine of almost every society that existed in a region where the climate would support the cultivation of grapes. Wine and beer often provide alternative beverages in areas where drinking water is not fit for human consumption.

In the examples I've cited, the use of psychotropic substances has a regular and recognized place in the social order. Whether as medicines, adjuncts to work, components of religious rituals, or elements of cuisines, many of these substances have been and still are consumed publicly and openly. They had (and have) well-defined places in the lives of the people using them, and, except for wine, nicotine, and perhaps beer, were usually not available in quantities large and inexpensive enough to support compulsive use.

I don't mean to say that excessive and socially unacceptable substance use was not a problem. There is evidence that hospitals which specialized in treating people with alcohol problems existed more than 5,000 years ago in Egypt. And belladonna and the related substances atropine and scopolamine, which are powerful psychotropic toxins, were widely used to induce sexual ecstasy (followed, conveniently, by loss of memory) in bacchanalian orgies and in witchcraft rituals such as Black Sabbaths. But substance abuse problems of earlier societies were significantly different from those of our own in one very important way. I can sum up the cause of the difference with one word: technology.

SUPERCHARGING SUBSTANCES

The problems I faced as a young physician trying to help my patients overcome serious substance problems went well beyond dealing with the controlled and socially acceptable use of psychotropic substances. My experience helped me understand that it's more difficult now than at any time in history to use substances in a controlled way, and that technology is at least partly to blame. New technologies have enabled us to do two things: dramatically increase the potency and availability of naturally occurring psychotropic substances, and create very powerful synthetic substances.

Within the past 150 years, these technologies have been developed to the point where today many psychotropic substances are available in concentrated forms that are hundreds of times stronger than the natural sources from which they are derived. In addition to being very powerful, they are potentially much more addictive than their natural counterparts. When they're ingested in concentrated form, their effects on brain chemistry are markedly exaggerated. In many cases, those using these concentrated substances often ignore, and even flout, the social conventions and legal restrictions that might otherwise control their use.

Among the earliest of such substances were the high-alcohol liquors made by distilling fermented beverages. Distillation of fermented drinks was widespread from the Middle East to Russia and northern Europe by the twelfth century AD. By the early 1800s in the United States, excessive liquor consumption was a problem that had begun to command the attention of doctors and moralists alike. This attention was certainly warranted: The per capita consumption of distilled liquor in the United States at that time was more than three times what it is today.

Liquor was only one of a growing number of concentrated addictive substances that became widely available in the nineteenth century. Morphine, the psychotropic substance in opium, was chemically isolated from poppy seeds in 1805. However, it was not until the invention of the hypodermic needle in the mid-1800s that a delivery system enabled morphine, which is still the most effective painkiller, to be used medically. Unfortunately, this new technology also enabled people to abuse the substance.

Cocaine, the psychotropic substance produced by the coca plant, was first isolated and extracted in the mid-1800s. During the last quarter of the nineteenth century in Europe and the United States, both cocaine and opium were widely available in tonics and patent medicines, and cocaine was an active ingredient in several soft drinks, and even in cigarettes. Cocaine was prescribed for the treatment of various medical conditions, from sinusitis to opiate and alcohol addiction. It was also touted as a cure for depression, while morphine was offered as a cure for cocaine addiction. The growing awareness of the substance's addictive potential was instrumental in the passage in 1906 of the Pure Food and Drug Act, which prohibited the use of cocaine in soft drinks and patent medicines.

Cigarettes provide another example of how the relatively controlled use of a substance can change through technology. Smoking was not a significant cause of widespread health problems early in the twentieth century, in part because most smokers had to hand-roll their cigarettes. Mass production helped change that. By offering packaged pre-rolled cigarettes, and thus making tobacco widely and relatively inexpensively available in an easy-to-use form, tobacco companies contributed to the dramatic rise in cigarette smoking in the United States and Europe. The development by tobacco companies of high-nicotine strains of tobacco, which has only recently come to light, worsened the potential for the abuse of nicotine through smoking.

The technology to extract psychotropic substances in high concentrations and the packaging and marketing of cigarettes and alcoholic beverages which contributed to the widespread availability of those substances are elements in the story of the rise of substance use during the past two centuries. The scientific and medical communities also played significant roles in this phenomenon.

THE ROLE OF SCIENCE AND MEDICINE

Among the most important components in the rise of substance abuse has been the role that science and medicine have played. By the middle of the twentieth century, the American Medical Association (AMA) was closely allied with the tobacco industry, and cigarette advertising presented in the pages of the *Journal of the American Medical Association* had become a very significant source of revenue for the organization. The AMA was one of the last major healthcare organizations to admit that smoking presented a significant health hazard, and its refusal to take a position against smoking provided an implied defense of the tobacco industry until well into the 1980s.

The creation of synthetic psychotropic drugs began in the 1920s with amphetamine, which mimics the effects of one of the brain's natural stimulants, dopamine. Despite the overwhelming evidence of serious and disturbing side effects, the medical profession has eagerly prescribed psychotropic drugs for the treatment of symptoms of all kinds. In doing so, it has contributed to the creation of an atmosphere in which the irresponsible use of psychotropic substances flourishes.

And flourish it has. By the 1950s, the earliest synthetic antidepressants, monoamine oxidase (MAO) inhibitors, were being used in the treatment of mental illness. Within a decade, the benzodiazepines, which include Valium, Librium, and Xanax, were being used to treat anxiety and induce sedation. More recently, serotonin-selective reuptake inhibitor (SSRI) drugs, including Prozac, Zoloft, and Paxil, and tricyclic antidepressants, including Tofranil and Elavil, have found favor among medical and psychiatric professionals for the treatment, particularly, of depression. Even more disturbing to me (and to many other responsible physicians) is the rampant use of psychotropic substances, particularly Ritalin, in the treatment of so-called ADD and ADHD, especially in young children. All of the substances I've mentioned here are very powerful, and all have the potential to be highly addictive. In fact, because they are so widely and indiscriminately prescribed, with the result that so many people develop problems from using them, prescription psychotropic drugs have become another class of substance for which treatment strategies must be developed.

THE FOUR MYTHS REVISITED

I've talked about the fact that late-nineteenth and twentieth century technology helped to usher in an era of supercharged substances of abuse. Unfortunately, society's strategies for dealing with the often devastating consequences of substance abuse have not kept pace. Several of the strategies still widely used today are based on outmoded "scientific" principles more than a century old. And those based on research done in the twentieth century often employ treatments that actually worsen the problems they are supposed to correct.

I call the three primary approaches that have emerged in the past 175 years or so the *moral, psychological,* and *medical/psychiatric* approaches. When they were initially developed, they represented society's well-intentioned efforts to treat substance problems, but their documented success rates in helping substance users recover are extremely low. These treatment strategies all perpetuate to some degree the four myths about substance use which I introduced in Chapter 1, and because they do, they often hinder rather than help recovery.

The moral approach to dealing with substance abuse started with the Temperance Movement in the early 1800s in the United States. While the influence of this movement has waned since Prohibition during the 1920s and early '30s, it continues to be an element of many treatment strategies. Equally as important, it remains a significant aspect of society's attitudes, particularly those of legislators and law enforcement officials, towards substance abusers today.

Those who have followed the moral approach see excessive alcohol and drug use not as biochemical problems but as problems of "character." In other words, character weaknesses of substance abusers are seen as the root causes of their problems. The moral approach holds that compulsive users are both responsible for their conditions and accountable for the consequences of their actions. Often, this leads to their becoming outcastes among family and friends, and to a withdrawal of support from the community and the workplace. Alcoholics and drug abusers were, and often still are, punished with jail or prison terms for their substance use. Needless to say, it was and is extremely difficult for substance abusers to overcome their problems under these circumstances, and the most negative outcomes are still the rule rather than the exception. Today the United States has the highest incarceration rate in the world, and studies suggest that more than 90 percent of those incarcerated are also substance users.

The 1950s saw the rise of what I call the psychological approach, with substance abuse problems coming to be seen by many as the result of mental, emotional, and social conflicts. The causes of substance problems were viewed as resulting from psychological circumstances well beyond the control of alcoholics and drug abusers, and those people were seen as not responsible for their conditions and not accountable for the consequences of their behavior. The psychological approach relied heavily (and still does) on counseling, and often involves psychiatric hospitalization. Both the moral and psychological approaches, while successful for a small minority, often result in a substantial waste of money and time, because they fail to deal with the biochemical factors underlying substance abuse.

I speak from personal experience when I talk about the failure of these approaches. In addition to my medical degree, I hold a PhD in Psychology, and psychological counseling has been an important element in my treatment of substance abusers. In one of the positions I held, as a physician and psychiatric consultant for the New York State prison system, I dealt with hundreds of drug users and traffickers who were serving prison terms. One of the things that became clear to me during that time was this: The very fact that so many people are in prison or on probation only because of their involvement with drugs is in itself a testament to the failure of the moral approach. It is a tacit admission that we have found no effective way to reduce or eliminate our drug problems other than to imprison so-called drug offenders, with the implication that character defects are in some part responsible for their plights. I can testify that most of the people I treated during this time were no more than victims of their own biochemistry, and the morality which put them behind bars failed to even admit that as a possibility.

My experience in the prison system also gave me insight into the psychological approach. My staff and I counseled many inmates with substance use problems. Despite the fact that they received very intensive and very competent counseling, within two years after their release, more than 80 percent of them had relapsed or were back in prison. I want to emphasize that I fully support psychological counseling as an important component in working through problems which are often associated with substance abuse. But I also want to issue this warning: Unless the biochemical imbalances which are the true causes of substance problems are corrected, the benefits of psychological counseling will be marginal.

But while the moral and psychological approaches have a fairly long history in substance abuse treatment, more recently, substance problems have come to be viewed as "diseases" in the classical sense of the word. I refer to this way of dealing with substance problems as the medical/psychiatric approach. One of my first encounters with this approach occurred while I was a medical student on clinical rotation in the Emergency Room at the University of Virginia Hospital. One patient was admitted on three separate occasions for serious gastrointestinal bleeding, a condition that is not uncommon in advanced alcoholism. Each time, after we had stopped his bleeding, sedated him, and stabilized his condition for several days, he was released with a prescription for an antidepressant drug. Most of the ER staff were familiar with him, and all knew he'd be back in a month or two. When I suggested to a staff physician that something should be done to address his alcoholism, which all those who worked with him knew to be the cause of his life-threatening health problems, I was told firmly, "If you want to be a social worker, you're in the wrong place. Our job is to take care of medical problems."

Now this physician's comment, which is representative, in my experience, of the profession's attitude toward substance problems in general, reveals a number of things. First, it reeks of arrogance. The doctor who made it was saying that until problems reached a critical medical crisis, they were simply not worthy of a physician's attention. They belonged to the "social workers." Unfortunately, both the arrogance and the lack of understanding characterizes many physicians' and psychiatrists' attitudes toward substance problems. Typically, when these professionals actually deal with substance problems, their approach is to treat chronic substance abusers as people who have contracted illnesses which are "caused" by the specific psychotropic substances which they use. Treatment for the "disease" of alcoholism or drug addiction under this approach is similar to the treatment of many other diseases, and often relies on the extensive use of drugs. Unfortunately, many of the drugs employed in these treatment programs are also potentially addictive psychotropic drugs which are supposed to offset the effects of or substitute for the original "problem" addictive substance.

Under the medical/psychiatric approach, the substance user is usually seen as a victim of a more serious underlying psychiatric disorder such as depression, much as those who get cancer or diabetes are seen as victims. Responsibility for addressing the condition at the root of the addiction is seen is seen as beyond the user's control, and recovery depends on the skill of the attending physician and the effectiveness of the drugs he or she prescribes to treat the underlying psychiatric problem, much as is the case with those being treated for cancer. Recovery rates are typically lower than 30 percent with the medical/psychiatric approach. Even more disturbing, however, is the fact that, while some of the drugs are beneficial in treating acute withdrawal symptoms during the first days of recovery, cross-addictions and brain damage resulting from the administration of prescription psychotropic drugs over the long term are frequent outcomes of treatment using this approach.

THE POWER RECOVERY PROGRAM

We're faced with a situation, then, that has three primary components. First, potentially addictive substances are readily available in highly concentrated forms. Second, the social and religious conventions which helped contain drug consumption in the past are often too weak to prevent widespread drug abuse. And third, by ignoring the nutritional factors underlying substance problems, traditional approaches to substance abuse treatment have undermined their own potential to help those in need to recover successfully.

In talking about the failures of traditional approaches to substance abuse treatment, I've brought out several problems with the attitudes and assumptions associated with these methods. Now I'd like to give you an alternative framework for understanding your own substance use, one which will enable you to avoid the impediments to recovery that are implicit in traditional approaches. I'll be talking about how my attitude differs from those of the approaches I've discussed above, and about how that difference, which is at the heart of the Power Recovery Program, puts the power to recover in your hands, enabling you to recover even if you've been unsuccessful in the past.

One of the first things you need to understand is how the traditional terminology surrounding drug and alcohol use is loaded with preconceptions, assumptions, and negative value judgments that can stand in the way of your recovery without you even realizing it. You'll notice, for example, that I rarely use the terms "addict" or "addiction." The term "addiction" conveys the idea of a permanent condition against which "addicts" must be constantly on guard. In almost all cases, this is simply not true. The Power Recovery Program can help you put your substance problem behind you. More important, after you've completed my program and have little or no desire to use psychotropic substances, if you experience nicotine, drug, or alcohol cravings, mood swings, sleep problems, or dysfunctional behavior again, you'll understand why you have them, and you'll know exactly how to correct the imbalances and eliminate the cravings by starting again to take your nutritional supplements.

You'll notice, too, that I generally avoid terms such as "chemical dependence" and "substance use disorder." These terms are very precisely defined in the fourth edition of the American Psychiatric Association's *Diagnostic and Statistical Manual of Mental Disorders* (abbreviated *DSM-IV*). And while having precise definitions of such terms may help a physician or therapist categorize and diagnose her patients' substance problems, it has very little to do with what's really happening at the biochemical level. Being "diagnosed" in this way tends to put you at the mercy of the judgment of a professional. More important, it is disempowering because it robs you of the means of recovering from a substance problem by putting the control in someone else's hands.

The Power Recovery Program does exactly the opposite. I believe that putting a diagnostic label on your behavior is self-defeating, unless you're in denial of the fact that you have a problem. I'm going to leave it up to you to decide if you have a problem and what you want to call it. To my way of thinking, there are three levels that you might find helpful in determining where you stand as a person who uses psychotropic substances. Are you a *substance user*? In other words, do you have a take-it-or-leave-it attitude toward drugs and alcohol? Or are you perhaps a *substance abuser*? Do you occasionally, or even fairly frequently, overindulge in the use of your drug of choice? Or, finally, are you a *com-*

pulsive substance user? Has the need to acquire and use a specific substance or substances become of primary importance in your life, often coming ahead of health, work, family, and friends on your priorities list?

It's not important where we draw the line that separates substance use from addiction. Diagnostic categories may be helpful to you as you take a look at the seriousness of your substance use and examine the reasons you want to bring it under control. What is important is that *you define for yourself the level of your involvement with drugs or alcohol,* and that *you determine to do something about it that is based on scientific research, something that truly works.* The Power Recovery Program, unlike virtually any other drug or alcohol treatment strategy, gives you the tools you need to bring your substance problem under control naturally, often without the need for direct professional intervention.

The Power Recovery Program will enable you to understand that, no matter what your level of involvement might be, your substance use is a *behavior* in which you engage in response to a specific biochemical condition or conditions. And I want to emphasize that, in a sense, it's a perfectly natural behavior. When you're irritable, unhappy, or unable to focus, you may turn to cigarettes, drugs, or alcohol for relief. It's really very similar to eating food when you feel hungry.

Using psychotropic substances is a natural and predictable response to biochemical imbalances that negatively affect your moods and behavior. With this in mind, remember that your focus in dealing with your substance use should always remain on biochemistry and not on the substance itself. And remember also that, despite the fact that substance use is one way to change the way you feel, the results, whether you see them as positive or negative, are only temporary. The surest way to feel good on a long-term basis is to balance your biochemistry so that you do not need or feel compelled to resort to using psychotropic substances.

CONCLUSION

We're entering a new age in dealing with substance use. It's an age based on our profound new understanding of the physiology of the human body at the cellular and molecular levels. It's an age in which our new understanding of brain chemistry will enable us to regain the natural biochemical balance we've lost. By doing so we can eliminate the need for psychotropic substances and in the process also eliminate the pain and hardship substance users and those close to them so often must endure. In short, it's the age of the Power Recovery Program.

3

Our Billion-Year-Old Biochemistry

What I discovered about traditional approaches and attitudes toward the problem of substance abuse in the early stages of my professional career was not simply that they were largely unsuccessful, but that in many cases they actually prevented people from recovering. This was an important insight for me as I worked on a new approach to the problem, an approach which would become the Power Recovery Program. But there were two other components that I had to integrate into my substance use treatment strategy before it would be complete. The first of these was biochemistry. The subject is somewhat technical, so I hope you'll bear with me as I take you through an overview of this important element of my program.

CELLS

I had majored in chemistry in college, and biochemistry was my favorite subject in medical school. During the mid-1980s, after postgraduate studies in psychotherapy and following training in family practice and psychiatry, my interest in biochemistry was rekindled. At that time, scientific research in the field was advancing at a very rapid pace. Important breakthroughs in our understanding of how the human body works at the cellular and molecular levels were being reported almost daily. The message this research was sending was becoming increasingly clear: Life is fundamentally a biochemical process, and any approach to treating substance problems which ignored that fact was doomed to failure.

All living organisms, from bacteria to plants to mammals, function according to very specific biochemical principles, and when these principles are violated, bad things happen. With this idea in mind—that the principles of nature were the foundation of all life and must be respected—I began to think of substance abuse as a condition which violated those principles in a fundamental way. As I learned more about the physical effects of disruptions of brain chemistry, I sensed that the answer to the problem of substance abuse could be found in restoring the biochemical processes according to the principles of nature, and that this could only be accomplished using natural methods.

When I renewed my studies in biochemistry, one of the first things I was struck by was the breathtaking enormity and complexity of the biochemical processes that occur at the cellular and molecular levels of life. Since most people don't really have any reason to study this subject beyond the high school level, we often don't become aware of the extraordinary miracles that take place at this microscopic level every second of our lives. I'd like to share with you this miracle as I take you through what I call *our billion-year-old biochemistry,* the foundation on which the Power Recovery Program is built.

The fundamental engine of life is the cell, and activity at the cellular level is the foundation of all life processes. The first cells appeared on earth more than three and a half billion years ago, and their appearance marked the beginning of the chemistry of life, which has blossomed into an enormously diverse catalogue of creatures. These natural biochemical processes have been tried and modified and tried again since the first cells appeared on earth, and they remain to this day the basis of all the activities of our lives. From apparently simple single-celled bacteria to mammals, the most highly evolved and complex organisms on the planet, activity at the cellular level governs all aspects of life. Yet, while they are extraordinarily complex mechanisms, which have the capability to design, power, and maintain all life processes, in almost every case cells are so small they are invisible to the naked eye.

There are as many as 100 trillion cells—every one more complex than any engine General Motors can even think of building—in each of our bodies. They function with unimaginable precision, working together to perform tasks as diverse as breathing and dancing and solving quadratic equations. A single cell of the relatively uncomplicated bacterium *e. coli* contains several thousand kinds of small chemical molecules, including more than 1,000 different kinds of protein.

Every one of the cells of our bodies contains more than 6 feet of *deoxyribonucleic acid,* better known as *DNA.* Each person's DNA contains his unique genetic code, the blueprint for all of life's biochemical functions. And each of us has more than 20 billion miles of DNA in our body. Within every cell, a myriad of life-sustaining activities is carried out. All of these activities take place simultaneously and constantly, and with extraordinary rapidity: Within each cell in our bodies, as many as 50 million chemical reactions and molecular changes per second are occurring at all times.

Each of our bodies' cells is enclosed by a flexible membrane. In addition to containing the contents of the cell and separating the interior of the cell from its surroundings, the membrane controls every interaction between the cell and its environment. One very important way in which it does this is by means of surface chemical receptors. Surface receptors enable the cell to recognize and respond to other cells and molecular substances around it.

An individual cell may have many different kinds of surface receptors, and there may be more than 100,000 of each kind of receptor on a single cell. They form a coating on the cell's surface, and they are in constant motion. Like seaweed responding to the movements of currents on the ocean floor, they continually monitor their environments for the particular molecular substances with which they are chemically compatible. Virtually all animal and bacterial cells are constantly engaged in the business of capturing and ingesting or responding to the molecular substances around them. These transactions take place extremely rapidly, often taking only a few millionths of a second to be completed. Millions of such transactions occur every second in most of the cells of our bodies. It is this capability of cells—their ability to recognize and take in specific molecular substances by means of surface receptors—that would provide an important key in my development of the Power Recovery Program.

The cells of our bodies are specialized, and each type of cell performs a particular task. Some, like muscle cells, form tissues and organs. Others, like certain cells of the pancreas, for example, manufacture and secrete enzymes which aid in the digestion of proteins. The specialized cells which are of particular interest in our understanding of substance use, however, are the cells of our brains.

THE HUMAN BRAIN

The human brain is an extraordinary aggregation of more than 200 billion specialized cells, called *neurons,* most of which may be capable of making up to 10,000 different connections, called *synapses,* with other neurons. So powerful is this organ that by some measures a single human brain has more raw processing capacity than the most powerful computer in the world. The primary functions of the brain are communications and control. Its neurons communicate within the brain itself and with other parts of the body to direct all physical and mental activity. But while the human brain is the ultimate messaging center, its cells operate according to the same principles as the other cells of the body.

Like other cells, neurons have chemical receptors covering their surfaces. Many of these receptors are designed to be occupied by substances called neurotransmitters. Brain cells communicate with each other by means of exchanging neurotransmitters, sending and receiving messages that govern every aspect of our lives. In other words, communication among brain cells is a *biochemical process.* Gaining a more complete understanding of how the process works was a key for me in the development of the Power Recovery Program, and I think it will help you realize the importance of brain chemistry in recovering from a substance problem.

When a signal passes from one neuron to another, it does so by means of neurotransmitters. There are two primary types of neurotransmitters: excitatory and inhibitory. Excitatory neurotransmitters generally begin or continue the process of message transmission in our bodies and brains. Inhibitory neurotransmitters either slow down or stop message transmission. In most cases, individual neurons are capable of both producing and combining with more than one type of neurotransmitter. The messages sent can be very dramatic and fast-acting—like the ones transmitted to our muscles when we're in a fight-or-flight situation and must act quickly—or very subtle and slow to take effect—for instance, when we're gradually relaxing before falling asleep. Dozens of different neurotransmitters have been identified, with each one influencing our moods, thoughts, and actions in different ways as part of the enormously complex physiology of brain function.

Because our brains are composed of so many cells, and because these cells are constantly transmitting messages involving many types of neurotransmitters, a continuous give-and-take among excitatory and inhibitory neurotransmitters occurs, with many factors influencing the kinds of messages that are translated into actions and feelings. For instance, when we're in a situation that requires high levels of concentration, such as taking an exam in school, our brains are called on to produce extra excitatory neurotransmitters to help us focus and stay alert. When we're getting ready to go to sleep, production of inhibitory neurotransmitters is increased.

In addition to being either excitatory or inhibitory, neurotransmitters are associated with a variety of moods and activities. Among other things, they modify and help us cope with pain and stress, they enhance our appreciation of pleasurable experiences, and they enable us to stay focused and motivated.

Like other cells of the body, neurons manufacture the substances they release by assembling them from nutrient molecules which we take into our bodies in the food and nutritional supplements, such as vitamins and minerals, we consume. You can think of this manufacturing process as a kind of biochemical assembly line. In this case, our brains require precise amounts of specific nutrients to manufacture neurotransmitters. If one or more of the necessary nutrients is unavailable for any reason, the cells of our brains are unable to manufacture sufficient amounts of neurotransmitters to enable us to function at peak efficiency.

Inadequate neurotransmitter production—which can result from insufficient nutrients in our diets—can cause dramatic changes in our moods and the way we behave. If nutrient shortages extend for long periods of time, mood and behavior changes can become intolerable, causing us to seek alternative ways to cope and to feel better. Shortages of specific neurotransmitters which control our emotions play a significant role in the development of substance use problems.

NEUROTRANSMITTERS

There are four neurotransmitters (or groups of similar neurotransmitters) which are of primary interest to us as we explore how and why compulsive substance use occurs and how it can be eliminated. They are: endorphins and enkephalins, two groups of structurally similar inhibitory neurotransmitters which are powerful natural pain relievers; serotonin, an inhibitory neurotransmitter that exerts a soothing influence on unpleasant emotions; gamma-amino butyric acid (GABA), an inhibitory neurotransmitter which helps alleviate anxiety and worry; catecholamines (kat-uh-kohl'-uh-meens), a group of similar excitatory neurotransmitters which help to govern our abilities to pay attention and to experience excitement and pleasure in everyday activities.

When our bodies are well-nourished, and when nutrients are well-supplied to our brains, we're able to produce these important neurotransmitters in adequate amounts. When we experience fright, anger, nervousness, anxiety, or pain in response to a stressful situation, our brains respond by producing greater-than-normal quantities of these substances. (For this reason, they're also sometimes referred to as *stress hormones*.) They enable us to stay alert, motivated and focused in the face of whatever has caused our distress. However, when we're unable to produce these neurotransmitters in adequate amounts, we often seek other ways to cope. That's where psychotropic substances come in.

Psychotropic substances work by mimicking the effects of neurotransmitters. This means that when a psychotropic substance reaches the brain, it is able to occupy receptors designed for a specific neurotransmitter, in effect fooling the brain into thinking that it is producing its natural neurotransmitter in adequate amounts. This temporarily helps bring about the effects that would normally be achieved by the neurotransmitters themselves. The four key neurotransmitters I've mentioned are critical to understanding substance use for precisely this reason. Because they play such an important role in the development of substance problems, I want to take some time to discuss each of them separately.

Endorphins and Enkephalins

Endorphins and enkephalins are our natural pain killers, inhibitory neurotransmitters which are overproduced by the brain in response, primarily, to emotional or physical pain and physical exertion. They function by occupying neurotransmitter receptors which would normally be receiving pain signals sent from other parts of the body. By blocking the transmission of pain signals, endorphins and enkephalins can enable us to continue to function even in the presence of physical or emotional pain which might otherwise disable us.

Imagine, for instance, that one of your ancestors, perhaps tens of thousands of years ago, was being pursued by a dangerous predator, and that as he was desperately running from his pursuer, he fell and sprained his ankle. If your ancestor gave in to the urge to stop what he was doing because of his pain, he'd quickly become a carnivore's dinner. To overcome this, endorphins and enkephalins, the brain's natural painkillers, would immediately have been produced in large supply in his brain, blocking his pain, enabling him to continue his flight, in short, saving his life. (Obviously, if he's your ancestor, his enkephalins must have worked.)

In physically demanding situations, such as athletic contests, our bodies greatly overproduce both the stimulatory neurotransmitters, which enable us to perform at high levels, and the inhibitory neurotransmitters, such as enkephalins, which dull the pain that typically accompanies extreme physical exertion. In addition to blocking pain, endorphins and enkephalins work together with excitatory neurotransmitters. While excitatory neurotransmitters function to make us feel "up," the ability to produce endorphins in adequate amounts makes feeling "up" a pleasant and painless experience. The euphoric "high" often experienced by distance runners is in large part the result of the release, usually following the point of exhaustion, of large amounts of endorphins.

The psychotropic substances that mimic the actions of the enkephalins in the brain include morphine, the potentially highly addictive painkiller derived from poppy seeds; heroin, the chemically altered derivative of morphine; and a number of prescription painkillers, including buprenorphine, Oxycontin, codeine (which is also derived from morphine), methadone, and Demerol. Alcohol also mimics the effects of endorphins and enkephalins. In addition to triggering increased endorphin production, alcohol can stimulate the production of the substance THIQ, which blocks out the experience of pain in much the same way endorphins and enkephalins do. To describe a drunk person as "feeling no pain" is accurate at the biomolecular level.

All these substances have chemical structures which mimic the shape of the natural painkilling substances our brains produce. Their structures enable them to bind to and occupy pain receptors designed to accept endorphins and enkephalins. But there are important differences between the natural painkilling substances produced by our brains and the psychotropic substances that mimic their effects.

The process of communication by neurotransmitters also includes a recycling (or "re-uptake") phase. After a neurotransmitter has passed along its message, it is often broken down or recycled to be used again. This provides a key to understanding how some psychotropic substances achieve their effects. Although the chemical structures of morphine and heroin are such that they can occupy endorphin and enkephalin receptors, these substances are chemically quite different from the brain's natural painkillers in all other respects. This means that they cannot be deactivated by the enzymes that break down endorphins and enkephalins as part of the normal recycling process. As a result, they occupy pain receptors for long periods of time, intercepting the transmission of pain signals and causing a numbing of pain and, in higher doses, euphoria and drowsiness. Although this makes them highly effective painkillers, it also causes them to be potentially highly addictive. In addition, it means that overdoses can be lethal.

Serotonin

Serotonin is another inhibitory neurotransmitter, but its effects are quite different from those of the endorphins and enkephalins. Neurons which produce serotonin originate in a region of the brain associated with the emotions, and serotonin is generally viewed as an *emotional relaxant*. Among other things, serotonin acts to moderate the effects of the excitatory neurotransmitters, preventing us from becoming overstimulated and irritable. Normal serotonin levels prevent us from emotional overreactions to difficult and frustrating situations. The inability to produce serotonin in adequate amounts can result in emotional burnout from frequent emotional outbursts and is among the primary causes of depression.

Among the psychotropic substances that disrupt the production, release, and reuptake of serotonin is a class of prescription antidepressant drugs called serotonin-selective reuptake inhibitors, or SSRIs, including Prozac (generic name *fluoxetine*), Paxil (*paroxetene*), and Zoloft (*sertraline*). These disruptions inhibit the normal serotonin recycling process, causing molecules which mimic serotonin to remain available to receptors for an abnormally long time. This keeps the receiving neurons artificially stimulated, temporarily increasing serotonin activity in our brains.

In fact, with continued use, SSRIs actually make serotonin deficiencies worse. The brain has many built-in mechanisms which enable it to regulate the production of neurotransmitters and maintain a state of mental and emotional balance. The effect of SSRIs in keeping receiving neurons constantly occupied by serotonin is to make it appear to brain cells that excess amounts of serotonin are being produced. In response to this artificial and unnatural stimulation, our brains can *reduce* their production of this neurotransmitter, making the problem of low serotonin levels even worse. In addition, much of the breakdown in neurotransmitters occurs in the junction between neurons, called the "synapse." If the serotonin reuptake process is interrupted and serotonin molecules aren't reabsorbed by the neurons which released them, serotonin stores can become depleted.

When SSRI use is stopped, symptoms of serotonin deficiency—including irritability, rage, compulsive behavior, and anxiety—return. Because the ability to produce and store serotonin has been further disabled by the SSRI drug, these symptoms are often worse than they were originally. In addition, within a very short time (in many cases as little as four or five weeks) after treatment with an SSRI has begun, the effectiveness of SSRIs often wears off. This, too, results in the return of symptoms, in response to which physicians often increase SSRI dosages. Because stopping their use can cause severe withdrawal symptoms, SSRIs are potentially addictive, and SSRI dependence can develop over time. One of the primary causes of the symptoms addressed by SSRIs—the inability of the brain to manufacture serotonin in adequate amounts—is actually made much worse through the chronic use of these drugs, because they alter normal serotonin production in our brains.

Drugs such as SSRIs are not the only substances implicated in the disruption of the serotonin cycle, however. Eating foods which are high in refined sugar—candy and cookies, for instance—artificially stimulates the synthesis of serotonin and temporarily elevates serotonin levels in the brain, often making us feel more relaxed and comfortable. If you've ever reached for a box of candy when you were feeling "down," you were—probably without realizing it—trying to find a way to increase your serotonin levels. (Other processed high-carbohydrate foods can have a similar effect, by the way, and I've often speculated that the relaxing effect of the serotonin increase they cause might be one reason high-carbohydrate diets enjoy such popularity. There's certainly little sound scientific research to support the claims of effectiveness that are made for these diets. (I deal with sugar/carbohydrate addiction in Chapter 9.)

Under normal circumstances, when we're asleep the pineal gland converts serotonin into melatonin, a neurotransmitter which is critical to normal sleep. Many substances and biochemical imbalances cause disruptions in the serotonin-to-melatonin production cycle. This often results in insomnia, especially the inability to stay asleep during the night, which is one of the classic symptoms experienced by many substance users and abusers.

Gamma-Amino Butyric Acid (GABA)

Like serotonin, gamma-amino butyric acid (GABA) is an inhibitory neurotransmitter associated with relaxation. GABA is instrumental in such actions as calming racing, worrisome thoughts which can interfere with falling asleep. GABA is also thought to play a role in preventing seizures and anxiety attacks, and GABA deficiencies are associated with chronic anxiety and panic attacks. So effective is this neurotransmitter that it has been labeled "the natural Valium of the brain." In fact, it should be the other way around: Valium should be called *the unnatural GABA,* because Valium can only *temporarily* make you feel the way you would if your brain were producing adequate amounts of GABA.

Because alcohol mimics the effects of GABA, many people often use it to unwind and relax. Another important class of prescription drugs, called benzodiazepines, also mimic GABA. These drugs, which are widely prescribed in the treatment of anxiety disorders, include Valium (generic name *diazepam*), Librium (*chlordiazepoxide*), and Xanax (*alprazolam*), among others. Both alcohol and benzodiazepines are potentially highly addictive, and using them, often for only short periods of time, can severely interfere with normal GABA functions.

Catecholamines

The excitatory neurotransmitters which are the primary focus of the

Power Recovery Plan are called catecholamines. The catecholamines are natural, all-purpose, go-for-the-gusto excitatory neurotransmitters. Dopamine and norepinephrine, the two primary catecholamines produced in the brain, handle separate parts of this energizing function. Dopamine regulates short-term activities, such as bursts of intense concentration, feelings of euphoria, and behaviors which must shift rapidly to accommodate changing circumstances. Norepinephrine, on the other hand, causes generalized, sustained alertness, helping us maintain a baseline level of awareness and vigilance.

Stressful situations cause our brains to over-release catecholamines. When we're in the midst of a stressful period in a relationship, for instance, or when the stress of our jobs is great, or when we're suffering from stress to our immune systems, we need *more* of the catecholamines to retain our focus and keep going. Our brains are geared toward producing short-term bursts of catecholamines, and when stress continues over longer periods of time, the resulting increase in the need to produce these substances can deplete our bodies of reserves of catecholamines and of key nutrients required to produce them. This in turn can limit our ability to produce and release catecholamines in adequate amounts to deal with new sources of stress, even after the previous period of stress has passed, causing us to feel tired and unmotivated, have difficulty concentrating, and have trouble experiencing pleasure.

Many people turn to stimulants, such as cocaine or amphetamines, to help them cope with stressful situations which require increased catecholamine production. Each of these drugs disrupts the dopamine cycle in a different way. Amphetamines, often prescribed as the drug Adderall for children diagnosed with ADD and ADHD, occupy dopamine receptors directly, mimicking the effects in the receiving neuron of dopamine itself. On the other hand, cocaine and cocaine-like substances such as Ritalin hinder the recycling of dopamine and cause dopamine to build up to abnormally high levels between neurons in our brains.

The four groups of neurotransmitters just discussed are among the most important chemicals in our bodies. Because they control how we feel, our ability to focus, and our energy levels, they're the keys to how we function in our daily lives. For these reasons, keeping them functioning at optimal levels naturally is vital to overcoming substance use.

DRUGS AND FRONTAL LOBE BRAIN FUNCTIONS

A critical location in our brains of the neurotransmitter activity associated with the use of psychotropic substances is the frontal lobe region. The frontal lobe area of the human brain, which is located behind the forehead and above the eyes, is considered by neurobiologists to be one of the last areas of the brain to develop, and it is the area which both enables and controls many of the capabilities which make us uniquely human. It is our frontal lobes, for instance, which enable us to predict what the consequences of our actions might be. In other words, our frontal lobes perform what might be called the "executive function." Because we have this capability, we're able to make the best choices based on the projected outcomes of actions we're contemplating and inhibit inappropriate choices.

But while our frontal lobes are critical in responsible decision-making, they also enable us to imagine the consequences of our acts for others, and by doing this they give us the ability to empathize. For us to become caring, responsible people requires that our frontal lobes be fully functional and unimpaired. In addition, frontal lobe functions, more than those of any other area of the brain, account for those characteristics considered to be uniquely human, including imagination, creative thinking, subtle humor, artistic appreciation and expression, our ability to empathize with others, and our ability to engage in psychospiritual activities, such as contemplation, prayer, and meditation.

Just as the frontal lobe area was one of the last areas of the human brain to evolve, it is also one of the last areas of the brain to mature and become fully functional as we grow to adulthood. It's not until we near the age of 20 that our frontal lobes are completely developed and functioning in ways that enable us to assume the responsibilities required of adults. Psychotropic drugs and alcohol not only impair frontal lobe functioning, they also disrupt the growth and maturation process of the frontal lobes in young people. For this reason, it is imperative that young people not use psychotropic drugs: Their use literally slows down, even stops, the development of the very parts of our brains that make us truly human.

CONCLUSION

Each of the healthy cells in our bodies knows exactly what it is supposed to do. None of them needs a doctor or a scientist or a psychotherapist to remind it how it is supposed to function. The only things our cells need in order to provide for us the biochemical foundation of excellent physical, mental, and emotional health are the proper nutrients in the right amounts and the absence of toxins that interfere with their ability to function properly. This is what recent dramatic scientific discoveries are telling us about our *billion-year-old biochemistry,* and it is for this reason that the nutrients I prescribe in the Power Recovery Program are so effective. The biochemical processes which are the very basis of life at the cellular level have been tried, modified, and perfected, literally for the past three and a half billion years, ever since the first cells appeared on earth.

The intricate and complex biochemistry that has emerged during that time has proven to be incredibly reliable and efficient. But its reliability and efficiency depend on biochemical balance, and any recovery program that ignores imbalances in these enormously complex processes is doomed to failure. The Power Recovery Program enables you to recruit nature as your most powerful ally by using natural nutritional supplements to rebalance your brain chemistry and help you stop your substance use for the long term.

4

Why Do Some People Develop Substance Problems?

I've talked about two of the critical elements in the development of my Power Recovery Program. First, because I witnessed repeated failures of traditional approaches to treating substance problems, I was able to understand that the very attitudes and concepts, even the terminology, which are integral components of those methods, often hinder rather than help the recovery process. Second, I was able to make the connection between substance problems and biochemistry. This led me to realize that biochemical imbalances, especially where they affect brain chemistry, are the single most important cause of substance use problems. I began to understand that many factors, including genetic vulnerabilities, poor diet, stress, and exposure to toxins, were at work to create the conditions in which substance abuse could thrive. It remained for me to discover how those imbalances could be corrected before I could fully integrate all the components of the Power Recovery Program. As it turned out, the incident which triggered that discovery affected me in a very personal way.

A PERSONAL EXPERIENCE

In my twenties and early thirties, I was bothered by periods of low motivation and lack of energy. While they weren't disabling, and while I was able to continue to function in spite of them, these periods of mild depression served to color both my view of life and my relationships with work and other people. I was fully aware that I was not getting the most out of many of the experiences that make life meaningful and pleasurable. I

53

knew I should have been enjoying my family and my friends and my work more than I was, but I didn't know why I couldn't. I was also aware that I often didn't have the energy to treat those around me with the care and respect they deserved. But I couldn't seem to overcome this pervasive condition, and I was beginning to be resigned to the prospect of living the rest of my life at the mercy of my moods. Observing some of these same traits in genetically related family members, I had decided to use heredity as an excuse, one unfortunately used by many other people.

In 1980, however, I experienced a life-changing event. I was a resident psychiatrist at The Upstate Medical Center in Syracuse, New York. At that time, a number of scientists and physicians were studying the use of nutritional supplements to treat psychological disorders, and one morning I happened to read two articles about clinical studies which reported success in treating depression with the amino acid tyrosine. I intuitively recognized the importance of this approach, and I went out immediately and bought a bottle of tyrosine tablets. Less than two hours after I took my first dose of tyrosine, my depression had lifted. Literally, for the first time in my adult life, I knew what it meant to feel activated and fully alive. Like so many other people who suffer from depression, I did not truly comprehend the difference between feeling down and feeling up. Not until I began to regularly take tyrosine, that is. In the intervening thirty years, daily doses of this amino acid—a safe, natural, and inexpensive nutrient for the brain—have prevented the return of my periods of low energy and absence of motivation.

I attribute the success of this treatment to the positive effect that taking the nutritional supplement tyrosine has on the production of the neurotransmitter dopamine. The amino acid tyrosine is one of the nutrients which is required by brain cells for the production of dopamine. By supplying my system with the tyrosine it was lacking, I was making the nutrient more readily available to the cells of my brain to produce this important feel-good neurotransmitter. They didn't let me down. My neurons began almost immediately to increase the amount of dopamine they produced, and my mood brightened as soon as this happened. I had discovered and corrected a chronic biochemical imbalance that was preventing my brain from producing the neurotransmitter dopamine in adequate amounts. Equally significant was that my personal discovery could be used by other people to change their lives as I had changed mine.

The personal release from the prison of low moods which I experienced by using the amino acid tyrosine was only the tip of the iceberg, as it turned out. More research was being done on neurotransmitters, especially their chemical makeup and the processes by which cells produce them. Two things were becoming clear: First, as with all molecular substances produced by all the cells of our bodies, nutrients are the only substances necessary for the manufacture of neurotransmitters. Second, we were discovering that other neurotransmitters in addition to dopamine have a profound effect on how we think, feel, and act. I myself can bear witness to the fact that, by increasing the amount of tyrosine available to the cells of my brain, I stimulated an increase in the production of dopamine which dramatically changed my life for the better.

UNDERSTANDING THE IMPORTANCE OF NUTRIENTS

My experience led me to expand and refine the use of nutritional supplements, such as vitamins, minerals, and amino acids, in the treatment of substance problems and mood disorders. Because it's central to the success of the Power Recovery Program, I'd like to go into detail about the importance of nutrients and how a variety of everyday conditions can contribute to nutritional deficiencies which cause biochemical imbalances. Throughout the rest of this chapter, I'll be focusing on three things: what nutrients are; how nutritional deficiencies are at the root of all substance problems; and why nutritional supplements are an indispensable component in overcoming substance abuse problems.

Let me start by emphasizing how critically important nutrients are. As far as our biochemistry is concerned, there are only two types of substances: nutrients and toxins. Any substance that cannot be used by our bodies' cells to carry out the biochemical processes that literally keep us alive is a toxin (or poison). In small doses, most toxins are harmless and can usually be "flushed out" of our bodies by our built-in toxin removal capabilities. In larger doses, toxins can impair cellular functioning and, if allowed to accumulate, can lead to death. (I'll talk more about how our bodies eliminate toxins in Chapters 6 and 17.)

Although the biochemical processes that are the basis of life are extraordinarily complex, the nutrient substances necessary to support these activities are relatively few. The trillions upon trillions of chemical molecules in our bodies, of tens of thousands of different kinds, are built from a very small number of nutrient substances. Apart from water, sunlight, oxygen, and fiber, which we require in order to live, there are six classes of essential nutrients for human life: amino acids, vitamins, minerals, fats, enzymes, and phytonutrients.

You'll notice that I don't include carbohydrates. While carbohydrates are relatively easy for the body to metabolize and are a usable source of energy, aside from a few kinds of carbohydrates called "glyconutritionals," which I'll discuss in Chapter 9, the vast majority of carbohydrates are not essential to normal biochemical life functions. In fact, the overconsumption of carbohydrates, which is mistakenly recommended by many physicians and dietitians, is one of the primary causes of many degenerative conditions that plague modern society. In addition, diets high in refined carbohydrates actually increase the likelihood of substance problems. I strongly advise almost anyone seeking to overcome a substance problem to cut down her intake of this nonessential food to an absolute minimum, and to increase the consumption of high-protein, higher-fat, nutrient-dense foods, including eggs, meat, poultry, fish, dairy products, beans, and nuts and seeds.

The fact is that most of us are not well-equipped to process large quantities of carbohydrates. We have inherited our biochemistry from our ancestors, who often lived for long stretches of time during a typical year without having access to carbohydrates. We would do well to emulate this behavior. (By the way, I'm speaking here of our hunter-gatherer ancestors. The development of agriculture began only about 8,000 years ago, not a long enough time for the dietary changes that came with it to have triggered dramatic changes in our biochemistry.) I'll have a great deal more to say about the negative effects of high carbohydrate diets throughout this book.

One class of essential nutrients, called phytonutrients or phytochemicals, consists of thousands of different types of nutrient molecules. A number of phytonutrients function chemically in the same way as certain vitamins, making them interchangeable as nutrients. Phytonutrients are found in virtually all of the plant foods we consume and are the subject of much current research, especially with regard to their disease-preventing capabilities. It is becoming clear that phytonutrients play essential nutritional roles.

The human body is capable, then, of performing essential life functions by combining and recombining fewer than sixty nutrient substances into many thousands of different kinds of molecules. Included in this list of nutrients are some two dozen amino acids, twenty of which are used in the construction of the proteins and enzymes that are the basis of all life. In addition, there are thirteen principal vitamins/phytonutrients that contribute to the healthy functioning of the human body, although a case can be made for many more. While vitamins and phytonutrients do not provide energy or serve as building blocks for other substances, they do function as co-factors and catalysts and are necessary to the regulation and completion of innumerable biochemical transactions. There are also as many as fifteen minerals necessary for the support of life. And there are six different fats, in the form of fatty acids, that serve as the primary sources of energy for the body and as immune system regulators. Fatty acids are also used in the construction of cell membranes and the myelin sheaths that surround nerve cells and in the production of neurotransmitters and other hormones. These nutrients must be made continually available in the proper quantities to our bodies' cells if they are to function properly and at peak efficiency.

RISK FACTORS FOR SUBSTANCE PROBLEMS

I've talked at some length about the fact that compulsive substance use almost always results from *biochemical imbalances which disrupt the normal workings of the cells of our brains.* I've expanded this idea by giving you an overview of how our bodies function at the cellular and molecular levels. Now I'd like to take a look at the four primary causes of the biochemical imbalances which are at the root of substance cravings and problem substance use, poor nutrition, exposure to toxins, stress, and genetic vulnerabilities.

Another way to think of these four "causes" is as "risk factors" for substance cravings, because the more prevalent they are in your life, the greater your risk of developing a substance problem. These risk factors, and the symptoms they cause, can continue for years after you've stopped abusing drugs and alcohol. It's important to note that the first three risk factors on my list—poor nutrition, toxin exposure, and stress—are present to some degree in almost everyone's life at times. In addition, each one of them is capable *by itself* of causing or contributing significantly to a wide variety of symptoms, some as obvious as heart arrhythmias, others as obscure and complex as depression. And where all three are present, they are often so intertwined with each other that it can be difficult to figure out which symptoms are caused by which risk factor.

Each of these risk factors can have a profoundly negative impact on your biochemical balance. In addition, they are the principal risk factors not only for drug and alcohol cravings, but for many other chronic degenerative conditions that are virtually endemic to modern society. And yet, they are almost completely ignored in most of the recovery programs of which I'm aware. The Power Recovery Program highlights the importance of these risk factors and provides substance users with the means to reduce or eliminate them. Let me take some time to discuss each of them individually.

Poor Nutrition

One of the keys to an understanding of the impact of nutrition on general health and on symptoms such as substance cravings can be found in the blood. Our blood is almost literally a "nutrient soup." After the food we eat is digested and absorbed, nutrient molecules are carried in the bloodstream to the cells where they're taken in through surface receptors and in other ways for use by the cells. Nutrient molecules which don't get into the bloodstream cannot be made available for use by the cells of the body. There are a number of reasons why this might happen, among the most important of which are that the nutrients are not in our food in the first place, we choose a diet of nutritionally-deficient foods, and our bodies have difficulty absorbing the nutrients in the foods we consume. In order to understand why, we need to look at the quality of the food we eat and at our dietary habits. Unfortunately, the picture is pretty grim in many ways.

The Deteriorating Quality of Our Food Supply

For the past fifty years especially, the quality and nutritional value of the food most people consume has deteriorated drastically. For starters, the tremendous increase in the use of pesticides and herbicides in modern agriculture has resulted in the contamination of much of our food supply with powerful toxins, which, because they become part of the food we eat, our bodies must process and eliminate. In addition, the soil in which plants are grown is no less a living thing than the plants themselves, and the use of pesticides and chemical fertilizers has contributed to the gradual deterioration of soil quality. The soil is being depleted of minerals and other nutrients that would otherwise be absorbed by growing plants and become part of the food supply. This has resulted in food with much less nutritional value than the food consumed by our ancestors only a hundred years ago.

Add to this the fact that a large percentage of the food we eat has been highly processed and refined, with much of the remaining nutrient content thus removed, and you can begin to get an idea of one of the primary causes of the decline in nutrition that is epidemic today: *The nutritional value of the food we eat has been significantly reduced in the past fifty years.* Many nutrients essential to healthy cell function which were part of our ancestors' diets are either missing entirely or in short supply in much of the food we eat. Obviously, if the nutrients are in short supply in the food we eat, they'll also be undersupplied to the cells of our bodies, increasing the chances of biochemical imbalances.

Poor Food Choices

A further cause of poor nutrition can be found in our eating habits, and no better example exists than today's high-carbohydrate-diet *fad.* Somehow the absolutely false notion that high carbohydrate diets are beneficial to humans has gained currency. Nothing could be further from the truth. Because the carbohydrates consumed in diets of this kind are often highly refined, and because so much high-carbohydrate food is relatively low in amino acids, this ill-advised diet alone can be responsible for biochemical imbalances which cause substance cravings in otherwise healthy people.

I'm going to give you a specific example of one of the many types of imbalances a high carbohydrate diet can cause or contribute to, but before I do, you'll need some background on the digestive processes that occur in the large intestine. There are more than 400 different types of single-celled organisms, primarily bacteria and yeast, which inhabit the large intestine. Collectively, they are referred to as *intestinal flora*. Several types of intestinal flora, including *e. coli, lactobacillus acidophilus,* and *bifidus,* are known to be beneficial. Others, including several varieties of yeast and many bacteria, can be very harmful. To put things into perspective, of the 200 trillion or so cells in the human body, upwards of 90 percent are single-celled microbes inhabiting, primarily, the large intestine, and they play a vital role in completing the digestive process and in maintaining biochemical balance in our bodies.

In healthy individuals, a balance is maintained among beneficial organisms and harmful ones. This balance is critical to the digestive process, for some of these microorganisms aid digestion by breaking down nutrient substances into molecules usable by the body. In addition, many of the substances they produce to defend themselves against other harmful microorganisms also contribute to our immune system defenses. When the balance is shifted in favor of harmful microorganisms, our immune systems must often produce substances such as antibodies and inflammatory mediators to counteract the effects of toxins these organisms secrete. While the complex interactions among intestinal flora are far from completely understood, recent research has made it abundantly clear that they are vital in the process of maintaining health and resisting disease. In fact, they are so important that disruptions of the "balance of power" among them may be implicated in conditions ranging from diabetes to cardiovascular disease to arthritis.

But let's get back to carbohydrates. Chemically speaking, the term *carbohydrate* is just a fancy name for *sugar*. Carbohydrate molecules are either simple sugars like fructose or are made up of two or more sugar molecules linked together into "complex carbohydrate" chains. By the time you've chewed that forkful of pasta or baked potato to the point at which you can swallow it, salivary enzymes have begun to break down many of those carbohydrate molecules into their component parts, and you're essentially gulping down a mouthful of sugar. As several experts have pointed out, eating a medium-sized baked potato is the equivalent of eating about half of a cup of refined sugar.

Now sugars are food for yeast. Yeast thrive and multiply on a diet of sugar, and what people call a high-carbohydrate diet is really a high-sugar diet. Because it provides the harmful yeast in our intestines with exactly the kind of nutrients they need, this high sugar diet can help yeast to compete more successfully against beneficial organisms in the large intestine. When yeast digest sugar, they produce alcohol, and alcohol kills many forms of bacteria. The alcohol produced by sugar-fed yeast in our large intestines kills off many strains of bacteria, including bifidus and lacto-bacillus acidophilus, which are beneficial to humans. Alcohol is, in fact, just one of many toxins produced by yeast in order to compete with other intestinal flora.

I've treated numerous people for problems related to high-carbo-hydrate diets, and I've found that a condition known as the *auto-brewery syndrome* occurs in many of them. In these people, yeast overgrowth becomes so serious that a miniature alcohol production center is estab-lished in their intestinal tracts. They're literally "brewing" their own alcoholic beverage. It can get so bad that they'll "blow" a .02 on a breath-a-lyzer test after consuming sugar. In other words, the yeast in their intestines are producing enough alcohol to raise their blood alcohol lev-els to just below the legal limit for driving a car, even though they haven't taken a drink.

Maldigestion and Malabsorption

There are other conditions besides nutrient-poor food and poor eating habits that can result in lower availability of nutrients in our blood. Pri-mary among these are *maldigestion* and *malabsorption*. Even if our diet con-sists of toxin-free foods of the highest nutritional value, we won't get the full benefit unless those nutrients are broken down properly and absorbed into the bloodstream and become available for use by our bodies' cells in carrying out life functions. Unfortunately, that's not always a given.

Digestion of food is performed by digestive enzymes secreted in the mouth, stomach, and small intestines. The enzymes at work in the small intestines are produced by specialized organs such as the liver, gall blad-der, and pancreas. Beneficial intestinal flora also assist in the process of digestion. Food is broken down through the process of digestion into its basic building blocks—simple fats, amino acids, proteins, and sugars—so that these substances can be reconstructed into essential molecules and body components, from enzymes to muscle tissue. Among the factors that can interfere with digestion are toxins, nutritional deficiencies, and the overgrowth of harmful microorganisms, such as yeast, in the intestines. Digestive enzymes, which are made from amino acids derived largely from protein, play such a critical role in promoting good health that I pre-scribe them as supplements for almost every patient that consults with me.

In healthy people, most digested nutrient molecules are absorbed through the walls of the small intestine and enter the blood or lymph to be circulated throughout the body for use by other cells. The internal surfaces of the walls of the small intestine are made up of billions of microscopic projections, called *villi*. These projections increase the surface area of the intestinal wall dramatically. In fact, the digestive tract of a healthy adult can have an internal area *equal to two tennis courts* through which nutrient molecules can be absorbed.

There are a number of possible causes of malabsorption, or a reduction of the ability to absorb nutrients after they have been digested. As part of the process of colonization, intestinal flora use glue-like substances to fasten themselves onto the walls of the large intestine. Where imbalances resulting in an overgrowth of harmful bacteria occur, they may literally outgrow their environment and force their way backwards from the large intestine into the small intestine. When they attach themselves to the walls of the small intestine, they can block off areas through which nutrients are absorbed. In addition, toxins from harmful bacteria can damage the cells of the intestinal lining, further preventing absorption. In some cases, this can result in the reduction of the area of absorption from its normal two-tennis-court size to the size of a small closet. And since about 90 percent of nutrient absorption takes place through the walls of the small intestine, anything that limits that absorption can have serious consequences for our ability to provide nutrients to the cells of our bodies.

Malabsorption of nutrients can also result from problems in digesting food completely. A variety of enzymes, produced by specialized cells and secreted, primarily, into the small intestine, complete the digestion of proteins. Digestive problems, such as the inability of the pancreas to produce sufficient quantities of certain digestive enzymes, can result in incomplete protein digestion. Undigested protein putrefies in the large intestine, becoming yet another source of intestinal toxin. In addition, undigested protein may pass out of the body in the stool, leaving smaller quantities of protein available to be absorbed and used by the body.

The end result of the consumption of poor quality, highly processed food, along with maldigestion and malabsorption, causes malnutrition. Malnutrition, in turn, causes starvation, a condition from which a significant majority of people in the United States and other western democracies suffer. And malnutrition can result in the brain's not being able to produce the neurotransmitters that keep us focused, calm, and happy, the key reasons most people turn to addictive substances.

Toxins

I've mentioned several of the toxins—including pesticides, preservatives, and chemical additives that contaminate much of the food we eat, as well as toxins produced by harmful microorganisms in our digestive systems and other systems—that can contribute to nutritional imbalances. Among the other toxins that most of us must deal with at least occasionally, and often on a daily basis, are prescription antibiotics and heavy metals.

Antibiotic drugs (the word *antibiotic* means *against life*) are powerful poisons. They're designed to kill bacteria that cause infectious diseases, and I'm the first to agree that antibiotics have dramatically improved the quality of our lives and lessened our risk of dying from infectious diseases. But antibiotics don't just kill harmful bacteria; many of them also kill beneficial bacteria that inhabit the intestine. This, in turn, makes them unavailable to compete with harmful microorganisms, causing or exacerbating imbalances among intestinal flora.

These imbalances are made even worse by the fact that most commonly prescribed antibiotics do not kill yeast. If, for instance, you take an antibiotic drug for ten days to get over a throat infection, you will have also killed large numbers of intestinal bacteria, seriously altering the balance of microorganisms in your large intestine, often in favor of yeast. And if you've had frequent antibiotic treatments, as many young children do today, or if you eat the meat of animals given high doses of antibiotics along with their feed, you may be at risk for chronic intestinal imbalances.

A high percentage of the grain and vegetable crops grown today is treated with extremely toxic pesticides and herbicides. When we eat such food, or when we eat meat from animals fed with pesticide-treated grains, our bodies must get rid of the toxins thus absorbed. When the toxic load is greater than our bodies can deal with, toxic substances can remain in the small intestine, actually damaging the intestinal walls, where most of the nutrients we consume are absorbed.

Among the other toxins which can contribute to biochemical imbalances and which are present in a high percentage of my substance abuse

patients are heavy metals. Mercury, lead, aluminum, and cadmium contamination can come from many sources, including dental fillings, cook-
ware, the water supply, and some of the foods we eat, especially deepsea
fish such as tuna and swordfish. These substances often compromise cell
functions in significant ways. The healthcare system today generally
ignores the threats to health imposed by toxins, electing instead to wors-
en the toxicity problem by overprescribing drugs, which themselves are
toxins, to cover up the symptoms caused by toxins in the first place!

Stress

In the previous chapter, I discussed how the over-release and depletion of
several specific neurotransmitters can be triggered by physical and/or
emotional stress. I'd like to expand on that by giving you an overview of
how both acute and prolonged stress can cause or contribute to nutritional shortages and toxin overload.

Among the first things our bodies do when we're confronted with a
stressful situation— whether it's as relatively non-threatening as a chance
meeting with someone we dislike, or as dangerous as nearly losing control of the automobile we're driving—is to begin the over-release of
"stress hormones." Our bodies' capabilities for responding to stress by
releasing greater amounts of neurotransmitters and stress hormones
greatly improve our chances of survival in true life-or-death situations.
However, our responses to the relatively benign stress that the majority of
us deal with in our daily lives are not always tempered according to the
seriousness of the situation.

In response to even relatively low levels of stress, the signals sent by
stress hormones cause our bodies to divert large amounts of oxygen and
glucose to the brain, muscles, and heart, which need to be mobilized in
stressful situations. Digestion, urination, and reproductive activities can
come to a virtual standstill during times of stress. In cases of chronic (or
long-term) stress, whether it's in response to an illness or an emotionally
or physically taxing event, the body continues to use larger-than-normal
quantities of many proteins and blood pressure remains high as we continue to deal with the source of stress.

High stress hormone and neurotransmitter requirements can quickly
tax our bodies' supplies of the nutrients needed for their production. In

extreme cases, and when stressful situations go on for long periods of time, our bodies divert nutrients needed in other parts of the body to the brain. During extended periods of stress, unless nutrient supplies are replenished and kept at high levels, chronic shortages can develop, leading to the inability of our brains to produce these neurotransmitters at the high levels required to enable us to continue coping. And because of the depletion of stress hormones, which also enable us to fully appreciate the pleasurable experiences of life, our capacity to experience the joy and pleasure that facilitates emotional bonding with others is also diminished.

Among the frequent results of unresolved long-term stress is what has come to be known as "burnout." People suffering from burnout (which is another way of saying "exhaustion") are often chronically irritable, angry, listless, depressed, and lacking in motivation. But in fact burnout is a chronic depletion of stress hormones and neurotransmitters due to a combination of nutritional deficiencies, toxin exposure (especially through the use of psychotropic toxins), and stress.

I've painted a pretty dark picture of people who are poisoned, starved, and stressed. The good news is that the Power Recovery Program will show you how to correct these conditions, whether you have a substance problem or not. But, while we can usually make changes to improve our diets and eating habits, lessen our exposure to toxins, and reduce the level of stress in our lives, when it comes to the vulnerability substance abusers have to psychoactive chemicals, there is one risk factor that we are unable to change. That component, of course, is the genetic component.

Genetic Vulnerabilities

It will likely be many years before we can do anything to directly modify any genes we may have inherited which make us vulnerable to the effects of alcohol and/or drugs. You've gotta be you, and there are no two ways about it. The genetic code which plays a significant part in determining who we are, biochemically speaking, is stored in the DNA in virtually every one of our bodies' cells. And among the functions DNA codes for are the several components of our responses to deficiencies in neurotransmitters caused by stress, toxicity, and nutritional deficiencies, as well as to the use of psychotropic substances.

While we can't change our genes, we can certainly understand the role they play in making us susceptible to substance abuse. What's even more important is that, contrary to what you may have heard, there's actually a great deal we can do to overcome the possible consequences of any such genetic tendencies we may have. The situation is far from hopeless. In fact, as you read this section you'll discover that even if you're highly genetically vulnerable, there is no reason you have to "give in" to compulsive substance use. And if you're already a substance user and have inherited vulnerabilities, I'll show you what you need to do to counteract your genetic tendencies and significantly reduce or eliminate your tendency to develop cravings for alcohol or drugs.

A majority of the studies which attempt to isolate genetic vulnerability have focused on alcohol, but even without scientific studies, most of us could identify friends or acquaintances who are genetically susceptible to alcohol abuse. Genetic vulnerability often surfaces as early as our teenage years, and it usually takes the form of someone who's capable of drinking heavily for long periods of time, often days, often with very little or no sleep. The person genetically susceptible to alcohol can often consume quantities of beer, wine, or liquor so great that they would make most people become violently ill if they hadn't already passed out. Those genetically susceptible to alcoholism also often react differently from the rest of us the morning after an evening of excessive drinking. Whereas most people spend the next day nursing deadly hangovers, vowing never to take another drink, those genetically vulnerable to alcoholism often find that starting to drink again is their key to feeling better.

When I speak of the genetic basis for alcoholism, and for other substances as well, I mean that there is a genetic *vulnerability* to nutrient deficiencies resulting from alcohol use and/or to exposure to psychotropic toxins (in this case, to alcohol). In animals, many genes associated with vulnerability to alcohol have been discovered, and it is likely that dozens more will ultimately be identified in humans as well. The more genes we inherit for these vulnerabilities, the more severe and rapid the progress any alcohol or drug problem we develop is likely to be.

Vulnerability to alcoholism has a genetic component, but that component simply translates into higher requirements for certain nutrients, such as amino acids and minerals, that support human life. In terms of brain chemistry, people genetically vulnerable to alcoholism process alcohol somewhat differently than those not as vulnerable. In some cases, this means that the alcoholic person produces higher levels of a toxic byproduct of alcohol called THQ, which works in the same way as enkephalins, the natural painkillers our brains produce. Other evidence suggests that alcohol artificially stimulates gamma-amino butyric acid (GABA). This artificial stimulation can result in an increase in the production of dopamine, the major "feel-good" neurotransmitter our brains produce.

Research also has also shown that in genetically vulnerable people alcohol can affect cell membrane flexibility and can influence brain cells' ability to manufacture and utilize the hundreds of enzymes that do the "housekeeping" of metabolism. These enzymes seem to adapt to the presence of alcohol and begin to function normally only when alcohol is present.

We have covered the four general areas that are considered risk factors for substance problems. You might be confident in your capability to change your circumstances when it comes to poor nutrition, toxins, and stress, but not so confident if you know or find out that you have a genetic vulnerability as described in the section above. The important thing I want you to understand is that, while we can't change our genetic makeup, we can work successfully through managing other aspects of our lives to minimize the potentially negative impact of many genetic conditions. When we work to reduce stress and the intake of toxins, and when we control our diets, we can go a long way toward overcoming genetic vulnerabilities.

CONCLUSION

In this chapter I've dealt with the risk factors for substance abuse, from the importance of the food we eat in maintaining the supply of nutrients we need for optimal brain function, to genetics, to such environmental factors as toxins and stress. These factors are the final pieces of the biochemical puzzle I've been putting together in Part One, and they will help you understand the key elements of your or your loved one's recovery.

Before you move on to Part Two, I want to reemphasize several of the ways the Power Recovery Program is unique, and why it gives you the best chance of recovering from a substance problem. It helps you to avoid falling prey to the four myths about substance use that can actually hinder rather than promote your recovery. It is designed to help you to get your body and brain back in synch with the principles of human biochemistry, on which it is based. It is a recovery program that addresses in a real and accessible way the true risk factors for substance problems and puts the "body" back into the recovery of body, mind, and spirit. It requires that you use only completely safe, natural nutrients. You can use the Power Recovery Program by yourself or as you're working with a physician or counselor, or if you're in a treatment program or a peer support group such as AA.

The Power Recovery Program puts the means to overcome the symptoms associated with substance use and to stop relying on tobacco, alcohol, and drugs *in your hands*. It shows you how to change the way you feel and behave without having to resort to psychotropic substances. I'll be giving you very specific programs of nutritional supplements that will help you to reduce or eliminate your substance cravings, detoxify your body, and correct the long-term damage your substance use may have caused.

Part Two

The Power Recovery Program

N ow it's time to begin the practical portion of the Power Recovery Program. You'll recall that in Chapter One I gave you an overview of the program's three stages: Quick-Start, Detoxification, and Long-Term Biochemical Rebalancing. Part Two will go into greater detail regarding the first two stages of the program.

Stage One, Quick-Start, is an initial program of nutritional supplements designed to increase the production of one or more specific neurotransmitters in which you may be deficient. I want to re-emphasize that even if you've been in recovery and have not been using drugs or alcohol for years, you can still benefit from all phases of the Power Recovery Program. Chapter 5 explains what you'll be doing in Quick-Start. To begin, you'll answer a series of questionnaires that enables you to identify the specific neurotransmitter deficiency or deficiencies that are most likely to be the causes of your substance use. Based on your questionnaire results, you'll purchase and begin taking several nutritional supplements, including amino acids, vitamins, and minerals, which will boost your neurotransmitter production and help you to reduce or eliminate your substance urges, mood swings, irritability, difficulty in concentrating, sleep problems, and other symptoms. That's all there is to Quick-Start.

Soon after beginning these nutrients, you'll be ready to start Stage Two, Detoxification. In Stage Two, you'll add another group of nutrients to your regimen that will help your body eliminate toxins. Many of these toxins have accumulated as a result of your substance use, and they can cause or contribute to your symptoms. Chapter 6 provides an in-depth discussion of the Power Recovery Program's Detoxification plan.

You'll actually be taking both your Quick-Start nutrients and your Detoxification nutrients at the same time, so Stages One and Two of the Power Recovery Program overlap each other. Each stage, however, performs a very specific function: Quick-Start is designed to restore disrupted brain chemistry and reduce or eliminate many of the symptoms associated with your substance use, while Detoxification strengthens your body's ability to get rid of toxic substances.

For many people, these two stages, along with a maintenance plan, are all that are required to be completely free of the symptoms associated with substance problems. That's why I've grouped the first two stages together in this section of the book, as well as included Chapter 7, which provides more information on maintaining your healthy status by making smart diet and nutrition decisions. Some people, especially those with a long-term history of substance abuse, may find that Stage Three, Biochemical Rebalancing, is also necessary. The third stage will be covered in Part Three of this book.

5

Stage One
Quick-Start

One of the most difficult obstacles you may encounter when you are trying to overcome a substance problem is how to deal with the symptoms associated with your substance use. As I've said, these symptoms can include everything from mood disorders to sleep problems to dysfunctional behaviors. This is because, during the early stages of withdrawal from nicotine, alcohol, or drugs, your brain has not had the opportunity to rebalance its biochemistry. It still "needs" the substance you've been using in order to compensate for impaired neurotransmitter function, and these biochemical needs translate into specific symptoms. And for many of you, even though you've stopped using drugs and alcohol years ago, symptoms that caused you to turn to substance use in the first place still persist.

This chapter, which guides you through the Quick-Start stage of the Power Recovery Program, will teach you how to rapidly reduce or eliminate the most common symptoms experienced by problem substance users. After a discussion of the specific symptoms for each group of substances and important background information on how the Power Recovery Program was developed, I take you through a series of questionnaires designed to help you determine which specific neurotransmitter deficiencies are at the root of your problem substance use. Based on your answers to these questionnaires, I recommend targeted protocols of nutritional substances designed to rebalance your brain chemistry and reduce your dependency on your substance of abuse. This chapter will enable you to design your own personal version of my Power Recovery Program and begin your recovery immediately.

SYMPTOMS ASSOCIATED WITH SUBSTANCE USE

The Power Recovery Program is a safe, proven, widely available method for reducing symptoms, especially during the early stages of substance withdrawal, but also if you're still experiencing the symptoms that led you to substance abuse even though you've been "clean" for a long time. In fact, I developed what I call Quick-Start to help enable people with substance problems to overcome this often difficult initial period of recovery. The information in the previous two chapters is critical to an understanding of how Quick-Start works, so I'm going to review it briefly for you here. This will give you a clear picture of why Quick-Start is so unique and so effective in helping reduce substance cravings and other symptoms.

A majority of people with substance problems use one or more of the following: nicotine, in the form of cigarettes or smokeless tobacco; alcohol; stimulants, including, primarily, cocaine, Ritalin, and amphetamines; sedatives, or "downers"; prescription antidepressant and anti-anxiety drugs; opiates, including heroin, methadone, and prescription painkillers such as codeine; and cannabinoids, in marijuana and hashish. All of these substances are *psychotropic substances,* meaning that they interact directly with brain cells to disrupt normal brain chemistry.

Scientific evidence strongly suggests that excessive use of any of the chemical substances I've listed above is almost always directly linked to a deficiency in the production of one or more of the four neurotransmitters I've mentioned previously: enkephalins and endorphins, GABA, serotonin, and the catecholamines, with the addition of anandamide, the neurotransmitter which is disrupted in those who abuse marijuana and hashish. Each of these types of neurotransmitter affects our feelings and behavior significantly, but they have widely differing effects from one another. If our brains are not producing enough serotonin, for example, we'll feel and behave much differently than if we're deficient in dopamine. When our brains are functioning normally, all of these neurotransmitters work in harmony, complementing and modifying each other's effects to enable us to feel and behave healthily. When the production of one or more of them is disrupted, our feelings can change, often dramatically, and our intellectual functioning, memory, and behaviors can be adversely affected. We may begin to look for ways to feel good again.

So direct are the consequences of neurotransmitter shortages that substance users typically develop recognizable "profiles" depending on which neurotransmitter they're deficient in.

Neurotransmitter shortages are usually associated with deficiencies of the nutrients our brains need to produce these critical chemical messengers. The Quick-Start stage of my Power Recovery Program works by "spiking," or significantly raising, the levels of a few key nutrients, making adequate supplies of them available to your brain so it can resume the production of normal amounts of neurotransmitters. Levels of the Quick-Start nutrients in your bloodstream remain high for four to eight hours after you've taken a dose of supplements, then they begin to dip, in much the same way they do when you go a long time between meals.

When nutrient levels go down, your brain's ability to produce neurotransmitters is lessened. This can result in a return of concentration difficulties, irritability and mood swings, and problem behavior. In this case, your need to use drugs to compensate for the underproduction may return. That's why, as you'll see, I recommend that you take the nutrients two or three times a day and avoid skipping meals: so that you keep the production of neurotransmitters at a high enough level to help ensure that your substance cravings won't return.

THE POWER RECOVERY PROGRAM

As I indicated in Chapter 1, the Power Recovery Program is a clinically tested and highly successful substance recovery strategy, and Stage One, Quick-Start, is one of the reasons for its success. Let me give you some more detailed information about my revolutionary program.

By the late 1980s, I had prescribed nutritional supplements in several hospital and rehabilitation clinic settings to successfully treat people with substance problems. In most cases, nutritional supplementation was one element in a program which also included psychological counseling and organized support groups. In cases of severe drug and alcohol abuse, prescription drugs were also used in order to help patients through the painful and often dangerous stages of early withdrawal. In these cases, after they began their programs of nutritional supplementation, patients were able to taper and stop the use of psychotropic prescription drugs much more quickly than those who did not take the supplements. Where the key nutritional supplementation protocols of the Power Recovery Program were used, whether by themselves or in addition to traditional recovery strategies, patients detoxified more quickly and generally experienced significantly reduced substance cravings during the early stages of recovery. Where they continued to follow the program of nutritional supplements after their hospital stays, the incidence of relapse was startlingly low. As mood swings and irritability lessened, sleep patterns normalized, and their ability to concentrate returned, they had less of a "need" to relapse.

As I've mentioned, in 1990 I was offered the position of Medical Director of Tully Hill, a fifty-six-bed, JCAH-approved (Joint Commission for the Accreditation of Hospitals) drug and alcohol detoxification and rehabilitation facility near Syracuse, New York. This proved to be an excellent opportunity to demonstrate in a controlled setting the effectiveness of the Power Recovery Program protocols, which I had been developing for the previous ten years.

Among the first things I noticed after I introduced the Power Recovery Program nutrients into the Tully Hill treatment strategy were the comments of patients and staff. Several times per week, counselors with extensive experience in the traditional approaches would speak with amazement about the rapid recoveries that seriously alcohol- and drug-addicted patients were making because of the Power Recovery Program methods. I'd hear comments like, "A week ago, I literally thought Mr. X might not make it. Now he's participating in aerobics class and openly expressing his feelings in therapy groups!", and "Mrs. Y told me that since she's been taking her nutritional supplements, for the first time in twenty years she doesn't feel depressed. And she's taken every antidepressant known to medicine." Several times per month I'd be the recipient of exuberant hugs from recovering cocaine abusers. These hugs would be accompanied by tearful outpourings to the effect of, "Doc, I started using crack two years ago. Since that time, until I started on your program, I didn't know what it meant not to have drug cravings. Thank you."

Frequently, perplexed patients and their families would ask me why they had to endure "wasted" rehabilitations that did not use these obvious and effective nutritional treatments. It didn't escape my notice that this question was asked by patients and their families, and by counselors, nurses and administrators, but very rarely by the other physicians and psychologists involved in treatment. Those who have vested interests in maintaining obsolete and potentially dangerous treatment methods (even though they are obviously ineffective) have come to dominate the treatment decisions in traditional rehabilitation facilities.

The fear and self-interest demonstrated over and over by those who fail to see the importance of including the "body" in a recovery of "body, mind, and spirit" is an old story, but it's one which keeps being repeated. I believe it's time for a new approach, one which has proven to be effective and which respects our bodies' abilities to heal themselves. It's time for the Power Recovery Program protocols to be incorporated into every substance abuse treatment program.

The proof of the effectiveness of the Power Recovery Program can be found in its results. A few years into my medical directorship at Tully Hill, we had perfected and standardized the Power Recovery Plan protocols enough to study and publish our outcomes. The study was conducted by New Standards, Inc., an industry watchdog organization. While the study measured several things, the results which point up the dramatic success of my approach are abstinence rates. Compared to clinical outcome study results for traditional approaches, the Power Recovery Program protocols achieve positive outcomes that are in many cases three times higher than expected.

YOUR PERSONAL RECOVERY STRATEGY

A recovering patient once told me that one of the things that made the Power Recovery Program so different from other programs was that it seemed to be designed specifically for him. Other methods, he went on, seemed to be asking him to fit a preconceived idea of what a recovering substance user should be. I found his insight to be very accurate. One of the problems with traditional programs for treating substance abuse is that they generally take a "one-size-fits-all" approach. The assumption seems to be that all alcoholics, for example, have the same "disease," and that therefore they should all be treated using the same drugs and counseling techniques.

Nothing could be further from the truth. The biochemistry underlying your substance abuse problem is unique to your body. In fact, although I've ordered in-depth biochemical profile tests for thousands of patients, I've never found two that were alike. You can accurately say that biochemistry is as unique as a fingerprint. Even other people who use the same substances as you do experience different effects from them and use them for different biochemical reasons. One of the distinctive aspects of my approach to treating substance problems is that it takes these differences into account. As you progress with the Power Recovery Program, you'll be designing a treatment strategy that is unique to you, one that is tailored to your own individual biochemistry. The Quick-Start stage is the first step in that process. Let me briefly review the steps you'll be taking to design your personal Quick-Start recovery program.

The first step in the Quick-Start stage is identifying which neurotransmitter disruption is likely to be a significant cause of your substance urges and other symptoms associated with your substance use. Another way of describing this is to say that you'll be identifying the specific neurotransmitter deficiency which is "primary" for you.

Each of the following four sections contains a case history of one of my patients followed by a discussion of one of the four key neurotransmitter types. Each section also contains a questionnaire for you to fill out. They incorporate the same questions each of my patients answers while I take a medical history at his first appointment in my office. Your scores on these questionnaires will enable you to identify the neurotransmitter deficiency which is one of the main causes of your symptoms.

Once you've completed all four questionnaires, add up your scores separately for each one. Your scores will help you determine which neurotransmitter deficiency or deficiencies are primary in your substance problem. When you've identified your primary neurotransmitter deficiency, you'll begin taking the Quick-Start nutrients to correct the imbalances that are causing disrupted production of that neurotransmitter.

You'll find the names and recommended dosages of the nutrients listed along with each questionnaire. I want to emphasize that the quality of the nutrients you take is very important. Using inferior quality nutrients can undermine the effectiveness of your recovery. In Appendix B, I've provided a list of responsible nutritional supplement vendors (see page 284).

Please note that in some cases, disruptions in the production of more than one neurotransmitter are at the root of a substance problem. Therefore, *it is very important for you to read each of the following four sections* and *complete all four questionnaires.* Although you can treat more than one neurotransmitter deficiency at the same time, if you do find that you're deficient in more than one neurotransmitter, you can first concentrate on treating the "relaxing" neurotransmitter deficiency, and then move on to the "excitatory" neurotransmitter. For instance, if you are deficient in both GABA (relaxing) and catecholamines (excitatory), consider first correcting your GABA deficiency. Then you can move on to the catecholamines.

As you've read, one of the keys to the success of the Power Recovery Program is that it recognizes that recovery does not depend on which substance you use but on which neurotransmitter shortages are causing the mood disorders, concentration difficulties, and sleep problems associated with your urges to use substances. Therefore the purpose of the Quick-Start questionnaires is to enable you to identify your primary neurotransmitter shortages and restore them to normal production. With nicotine and marijuana (*cannabinis* or *cannabinoids*), however, the situation is somewhat different. If you're trying to stop using cigarettes, smokeless tobacco, or marijuana, *and you don't have a problem with any other substances,* you can skip over the following questionnaires and go directly to one of the sections near the end of this chapter entitled "Quick-Start for Smokers" or "Quick-Start for Marijuana Users." Begin taking the nutrients recommended in the section that deals with your problem substance. Then proceed to Stage Two in Chapter 6 and begin taking your detoxification nutrients.

If you have problems with nicotine or cannabinoids *and* one or more other substances, however, you should first answer the questionnaires, then take the recommended nutrients based on your questionnaire answers. For instance, if you abuse cocaine and alcohol in addition to cigarettes or marijuana, and your questionnaire answers indicate that you are deficient in catecholamines and serotonin, you should take the nutritional supplements prescribed to correct those deficiencies. In this case, you'd want to first treat your serotonin deficiency, then deal with your catecholamine deficiency, then tackle your smoking problem. You may find that the nutritional supplements you take for serotonin and catecholamines will also curb your desire for cigarettes or marijuana. After you've got your other substance problem or problems under control, you can return to the Quick-Start for Smokers or Quick-Start for Marijuana Users plan if you still need to deal with either of these problems.

IS A SEROTONIN DEFICIENCY CAUSING YOUR SUBSTANCE ABUSE PROBLEM?

Joyce D. is a 38-year-old mother of three. She works part-time, and she and her husband have been married for thirteen years. They have two daughters, ages 7 and 9, and one son, age 5. Joyce had been seeing a psychotherapist for several years in an attempt to deal with her "anger issues." She described herself as "irritable all the time" and having "little patience with people." She explained that the only way she'd been able to keep her anger under control was with the medications her doctors had prescribed and with alcohol. Joyce also indicated that she often craved sweets and that she frequently woke up during the night and had difficulty getting back to sleep.

During most of our first interview, Joyce looked away from me. When speaking about something that hit close to home, such as her deteriorating relationship with her daughters, she often wrung her hands. "Excuse my language, but sometimes I can just be such a bitch," she said. Joyce had begun drinking in secret about six years ago. When her husband found out, he was sympathetic and suggested she get help. After three months of psychotherapy, her symptoms remained. Her family doctor had prescribed many antidepressants, including Prozac, Effexor, Paxil, and Zoloft. These seemed to offer temporary relief, but she would experience intense side effects when she tried to stop taking her medications. She continued to drink in private along with taking her medications, a very dangerous practice, but though her husband, therapist, and family doctor knew she was drinking, they said nothing.

Joyce knew that alcohol and prescription drugs were robbing her of a close relationship with her children. "It feels like I'm not really a part of their lives. Oh, I'm there, but I'm missing out on something, I know it. That closeness, if you know what I mean. That's supposed to be there between a mother and her children. I mean, if alcohol and prescription drugs are the only things that make me functional, what good am I? What kind of life is that? I keep thinking, 'There's got to be a better way.' No, I should say, 'I know there's a better way.' And I've just got to find it." Her depression, characterized by anger, irritability, and sleep problems, along with the fact that she got some relief from her symptoms when she abused sugar and alcohol and took antidepressants, help to identify Joyce as a serotonin-deficient substance abuser.

Serotonin is produced by neurons primarily from the amino acid tryptophan and several vitamins and minerals. Serotonin is manufactured during the day by means of a multi-step production process. In the final step of this process, melatonin, a neurotransmitter that is crucial to normal sleep, is made from serotonin. Alcohol abuse often masks deficiencies in serotonin production.

Serotonin Deficiency Questionnaire

The questionnaire on page 80 will enable you to find out whether a disruption in the production of serotonin is primary in your substance use problem. Remember, even if your profile seems very different from Joyce's, you should go ahead and fill in the following questionnaire. Your score will help you determine if you are serotonin-deficient.

Essential Nutrients for Overcoming Serotonin Deficiency

If your scores on the questionnaire on page 80 indicate that you are either *probably* or *very probably* serotonin-deficient, a disruption in the production of serotonin is very likely primary in your substance use problem. Listed below you will find the essential nutrients you should take to correct the nutritional deficiencies that are at the root of your serotonin deficiency. Purchase these nutrients and begin taking them in the recommended doses as soon as possible. This should reduce or eliminate your substance urges and other symptoms within twenty-four to seventy-two hours. Please note that in Appendix B, which begins on page 284 I've given some tips on how and where to purchase nutrients.

Take the following nutrients to address your core nutrient shortages if your questionnaire score indicates that a serotonin deficiency might be primary in your substance abuse problem:

5HTP (5 hydroxytryptophan): Up to 300 milligrams (mg), three times daily, one hour before breakfast and dinner, and at bedtime. Begin with 100 mg twice per day, as that may be sufficient to enable you to restore your sero-

SEROTONIN DEFICIENCY QUESTIONNAIRE

If you answer "yes" to any of the following questions, enter the number of points indicated in the blank space to the right. Enter 0 (zero) if you answer "no."

1. Is alcohol your drug of choice? *If yes, 3 points.* _____

2. If you have used marijuana, does it have a relaxing effect on you? *If yes, 2 points.* _____

3. Have you ever obtained relief from symptoms of depression by taking prescription antidepressants, such as Prozac, Paxil, or Zoloft? *If yes, 5 points.* _____

4. Have you ever gotten relief from your symptoms by taking 5HTP or the amino acid tryptophan? *If yes, 5 points.* _____

5. Does eating high-sugar foods or processed carbohydrates relax you and/or relieve your irritability and anger? *If yes, 4 points.* _____

6. Do you often have the sense that you're "out of sync" or not attuned to what's going on around you, and that a few drinks gets you "reconnected?" *If yes, 2 points.* _____

7. Do you have a history of angry and irritable depression? *If yes, 2 points.* _____

8. Do you have a regular pattern of unexplained rages or a history of explosive or assaultive behavior? *If yes, 3 points.* _____

9. Do you have a history of sleep problems, especially waking up early and not being able to get back to sleep? *If yes, 2 points.* _____

10. Is there a history of depression in your family? *If yes, 2 points.* _____

11. Do you often experience symptoms of gastrointestinal distress, including gas, bloating, loose stools, constipation, and/or abdominal discomfort? *If yes, 3 points.* _____

    Total _____

Total of 12 to 15 points: You are *probably* serotonin-deficient.

Total of 16 or more points: You are *very probably* serotonin-deficient.

tonin levels. If that's not enough, slowly work your way up to 300 mg in each dose by adding, every three or four days, 100 mg to each dose.

Tryptophan, an amino acid, is the primary nutrient required by neurons to produce serotonin, and it can be used in place of 5HTP. 5HTP is made from tryptophan during the serotonin production cycle, and 5HTP is about ten times stronger than tryptophan, so it will help you restore your serotonin levels more quickly than tryptophan. Some people, however, respond better to tryptophan than to 5HTP, although the reasons for this are unknown. Tryptophan and 5HTP can be taken together. (Note: If you are taking antidepressant medication, you should consult with a healthcare professional before taking 5HTP or tryptophan.)

L-Glutamine: Up to 1,000 mg, four times daily, one hour before meals and at bedtime. Glutamine is an amino acid that helps in relaxation and helps raise low blood sugar levels. It is available in tablet and powder form. (The powder is less expensive). Please note that if you have cirrhosis of the liver or severe liver disease, you should consult with a healthcare professional before taking glutamine.

B-Complex Vitamin Capsule, or Multi-Vitamin with High Levels of B Vitamins: At least one capsule, three times daily, with 5HTP or tryptophan. Vitamin B_3 (niacin), folic acid, vitamin B_6 (pyridoxine), vitamin C, iron, and copper are all required for the production of serotonin. Your B-vitamin tablet should contain at least 50 mg of vitamins B_3 and B_6, but you should take less than 300 mg per day of each.

To avoid "niacin flush," an unpleasant reddening and sensitivity of the skin from too much niacin, make sure the niacin in your B-vitamin supplement is in the form of niacinamide or inositol hexaniacinate. Your B-vitamin capsule should also contain at least 400 mcg of folic acid, and it's okay to take up to 1,000 mcg, or 1 mg, of this vitamin. Please note that taking a B-vitamin supplement may make your urine bright yellow. This is perfectly normal and is a result of your body's elimination of B vitamins which it can't use.

Vitamin C: At least 500 mg, three times daily. Vitamin C is another important cofactor in the production of serotonin, and up to 5,000 mg per day can safely be taken. Please note that large doses of vitamin C may cause loose bowel movements. If this occurs, reduce your vitamin C dosage until you resume normal bowel movements.

Multi-Mineral Supplement: The minerals you need may be included in a multi-vitamin, multi-mineral supplement. If you choose to take a separate mineral supplement, make sure it contains the following, and take enough tablets each day to roughly equal the following dosages: calcium, 1,000 mg; magnesium, 300 mg; potassium, 100 mg; iron, 20 mg; zinc, 20 mg; manganese, 6 mg; chromium, 400 mcg; selenium, 60 mcg; molybdenum, 50 mcg.

Chromium is especially important to serotonin-deficient people because it helps serotonin work at serotonin receptors. It is important that you not supplement with copper if you're serotonin-deficient. If you do take a supplement with copper, you'll need to take extra zinc to counteract the fact that copper excess can block the synthesis of serotonin by neurons. Please note that if you are receiving dialysis treatments or have severe kidney disease, you should consult with a healthcare professional before taking mineral supplements.

You'll want to take your Quick-Start serotonin supplements for at least four weeks, and probably several weeks more, depending on your results. Monitor how you feel and behave, and consult with others around you for additional input as to how you're progressing. I'm confident you'll find you're making remarkable progress during this stage of your personal Power Recovery Program.

IS A GABA DEFICIENCY AT THE ROOT
OF YOUR SUBSTANCE ABUSE PROBLEM?

Marilyn S. was 77 years old when she first came to see me. Since the death of her husband more than two years earlier, she had been depressed, panicky, and anxious, and had experienced difficulty falling asleep. She explained that she just didn't want to get out of bed in the morning, and, although she had always been an active gardener, she had even let her gardening activities slide. Her daughter lived out of state, and, though they talked on the phone twice per week, Marilyn didn't want to burden her daughter with her problems. She felt sure her depression would lift after the shock of her husband's death wore off. In the meantime, she had begun drinking. Alcohol seemed to help her cope with her feelings of anxiety and fear.

A family friend who had been through a period of anxiety and panic herself gave Marilyn some Valium tablets, and they made her feel much better. "I know you shouldn't take someone else's prescription," she said, "but what harm could it do?" When she had used up the Valium her friend gave her, she asked her family physician of more than forty years to give her a prescription for the drug, which he did. The Valium worked fine for a few weeks, but then her symptoms returned and she began to drink even more heavily to suppress them. "Even though I didn't feel like getting out of bed in the morning, I just couldn't seem to go to sleep at night without using alcohol," she said.

GABA Deficiency Questionnaire

Marilyn's profile is typical of someone with a GABA-related deficiency. GABA is produced by neurons from the amino acid glutamate in the presence of vitamin B_6. The questionnaire on page 84 will enable you to find out whether disruptions in the production of GABA are primary in your substance use problem. Remember that Marilyn's case history is just one example of how GABA deficiencies can develop and cause chemical dependencies. Even if your profile seems very different from Marilyn's, you should go ahead and fill in the following questionnaire. Your score will help you determine if you are GABA-deficient.

Essential Nutrients for Overcoming GABA Deficiency

If your scores on the questionnaire on page 84 indicate that you are either *probably* or *very probably* GABA-deficient, the essential nutrients you should take to correct this problem are listed below. Purchase these nutrients and begin taking them in the recommended doses as soon as possible. This should reduce or eliminate your substance urges and other symptoms within twenty-four to seventy-two hours. Please note that in Appendix B, which begins on page 284, I've given some tips on how and where to purchase nutrients.

GABA DEFICIENCY QUESTIONNAIRE

If you answer "yes" to any of the following questions, enter the number of points indicated in the blank space to the right. Enter 0 (zero) if you answer "no."

1. Are sedatives, sleeping pills, or "downers" your drug of choice? *If yes, 5 points.* _____

2. Is alcohol your drug of choice? *If yes, 2 points.* _____

3. Does alcohol relax you or help you to sleep? *If yes, 4 points.* _____

4. Have you ever obtained relief from symptoms of anxiety by taking prescription drugs such as Ativan, Klonopin, Valium, or Xanax, or by taking sedatives? *If yes, 5 points.* _____

5. Do you often have symptoms such as headache, irritability, and/or dizziness when you go four hours or more without food? *If yes, 5 points.* _____

6. Do you have a history of panic attacks or severe anxiety? *If yes, 3 points.* _____

7. Do you have a tendency to be thin or underweight? *If yes, 2 points.* _____

8. Do you have problems sleeping, especially falling asleep? *If yes, 2 points.* _____

9. Do you have sugar cravings? *If yes, 2 points.* _____

10. Is there a history of anxiety or panic disorder in your family? *If yes, 2 points.* _____

Total _____

Total of 12 to 15 points: You are *probably* GABA-deficient.

Total of 16 or more points: You are *very probably* GABA-deficient.

Take the following primary nutrients if you are GABA-deficient:

L-Glutamine: Up to 3,500 mg (about one heaping teaspoonful of glutamine powder), four times daily, one hour before breakfast, lunch, and dinner, and at bedtime. You may begin with 1,500 mg, twice per day, and work up to the recommended dosage, if you like. Glutamine is an amino acid required for GABA production. It is available in tablet and powder form (powder is less expensive). Please note that if you have cirrhosis of the liver or severe liver disease, you should consult with a healthcare professional before taking glutamine.

GABA: Up to 1,000 mg, three times per day. Some GABA-deficient people, especially those who are genetically predisposed to under-produce GABA, find that they derive the greatest benefit from taking GABA directly, instead of glutamine. If you find that taking glutamine doesn't produce positive results, you might want to try taking GABA. Also, you can elect to take both GABA and glutamine, if you'd like, with no ill effects.

L-Taurine: Up to 1,000 mg with each dose of glutamine. Taurine is another "relaxing" amino acid, and it assists the mineral magnesium in getting into our cells.

B-Complex Vitamin Capsule, or Multi-Vitamin with High Levels of B Vitamins: At least one capsule, three times daily, with glutamine. Vitamin B_3 (niacin), folic acid, vitamin B_6 (pyridoxine), vitamin C, iron, and copper are all required for the production of GABA. Your B-vitamin tablet should contain at least 50 mg of vitamins B_3 and B_6, but you should take less than 300 mg per day of each.

To avoid "niacin flush," an unpleasant reddening and sensitivity of the skin from too much niacin, make sure the niacin in your B-vitamin supplement is in the form of niacinamide or inositol hexaniacinate. Your B-vitamin capsule should also contain at least 400 mcg of folic acid, and it's okay to take up to 1,000 mcg, or 1 mg, of this vitamin. Please note that taking a B-vitamin supplement may make your urine bright yellow. This is perfectly normal and is a result of your body's elimination of B vitamins which it can't use.

Vitamin C: At least 500 mg, three times daily. Vitamin C is another important cofactor in the production of GABA, and up to 5,000 mg per day can safely be taken. Please note that large doses of vitamin C may cause loose bowel movements. If this occurs, reduce your vitamin C dosage until you resume normal bowel movements.

Multi-Mineral Supplement: The minerals you need may be included in a multi-vitamin, multi-mineral supplement. If you choose to take a separate mineral supplement, however, make sure it contains the following, and take enough tablets each day to roughly equal the following dosages: calcium, 1,000 mg; magnesium, 300 mg; potassium, 100 mg; iron, 20 mg; zinc, 20 mg; manganese, 6 mg; chromium, 400 mcg; selenium, 60 mcg; molybdenum, 50 mcg.

Magnesium is very important in GABA deficiencies, because it is necessary for the brain to be able to synthesize GABA. You'll notice that the mineral copper is not on the list above. It is important for GABA-deficient people to avoid supplementing with copper if possible. If your mineral supplements do contain copper, it is important that they also contain zinc, which helps to keep the copper in the correct balance. Please note that if you are receiving dialysis treatments or have severe kidney disease, you should consult with a healthcare professional before taking mineral supplements.

You'll want to take your Quick-Start GABA supplements for at least four weeks, and probably several weeks more, depending on your results. Monitor how you feel and behave, and consult with others around you for additional input as to how you're progressing. I'm confident you'll find you're making remarkable progress during this stage of your personal Power Recovery Program.

ARE YOU AN ENDORPHIN/ENKEPHALIN-DEFICIENT SUBSTANCE ABUSER?

During my first interview with Bill W., he described himself as a "40-year-old workaholic." Bill owns his own construction business, and it's not unusual for him to put in eighty- and ninety-hour weeks at his office. He frequently experienced severe back pain. As he put it, "I'm a hands-on boss. I like to get out to each of our different sites at least once a week to see how things are going with my own eyes." He dated his recurring back pain to an incident that occurred two years ago when, in his words, "I got a little bit impatient at one of the jobs and tried to move a piece of equipment that I should have left to one of the crew." X-rays revealed a bulging disc in his lower back, and his doctor prescribed at least two weeks of bedrest and the painkiller Darvon. "Two weeks in bed," Bill laughed. "It just wasn't going to happen."

Bill had always been something of a drinker. "Even before the injury it seemed like I used to get headaches a lot," he told me. "Drinking just seemed to help ease the pain for a while, and it helped me unwind." Bill was also, in his words, "an aspirin junkie." Often he would take from twelve to fifteen aspirin tablets to help himself get through the day. Since his back injury, Bill had become cross-addicted to the powerful painkiller Oxycontin. His difficulties in dealing with severe back pain help identify Bill as a classic endorphin/enkephalin-deficient substance abuser. Endorphin/enkephalin-deficient people like Bill often turn to opiates to relieve their distress.

The amino acid DL-phenylalanine is helpful in restoring normal enkephalin levels because it slows down the action of enzymes which deactivate them. This enables enkephalins to occupy receptors and block pain impulses for longer-than-normal periods, thereby restoring their painkilling effects.

Endorphin/Enkephalin Deficiency Questionnaire

The questionnaire on page 88 will help you determine whether disruptions in the production of endorphins and enkephalins are primary in your substance use problem. Again, keep in mind that Bill's case history is just one example of the ways endorphin and enkephalin deficiencies can develop and cause chemical dependencies. Even if your profile seems very different from Bill's, you should go ahead and fill in the following questionnaire. Your score will help you determine if you are deficient in endorphins and enkephalins.

Essential Nutrients for Overcoming an Endorphin/Enkephalin Deficiency

If your scores on the questionnaire on page 88 indicate that you are either *probably* or *very probably* endorphin-deficient, the essential nutrients you should take to correct this problem are listed below. Purchase these nutrients and begin taking them in the recommended doses as soon as possible. If you're currently using opioids, this should help reduce or eliminate your need to use them within twenty-four to seventy-two hours. If you suffer from PTSD, these supplements can greatly improve your chances of

ENDORPHIN/ENKEPHALIN DEFICIENCY QUESTIONNAIRE

If you answer "yes" to any of the following questions, enter the number of points indicated in the blank space to the right. Enter 0 (zero) if you answer "no."

1. Are heroin, Darvon, codeine, methadone Oxycontin, and/or other opiates such as heroin your drugs of choice? *If yes, 5 points.* _____

2. Have you ever had difficulty stopping the use of painkilling drugs such as codeine, Darvon, methadone, or other opioids? *If yes, 3 points.* _____

3. Do you use drugs or alcohol to carve out a respite or "time out" from a very busy, active life? *If yes, 4 points.*_____

4. Have you ever been diagnosed with Post-Traumatic-Stress Disorder (PTSD)? *If yes, 5 points.* _____

5. Are you troubled by chronic pain, such as back pain, headaches, etc.? *If yes, 1 point.* _____

6. Do you have difficulty enjoying pleasurable experiences much of the time (and not just when you're feeling down)? *If yes, 1 point.* _____

7. Do you have low pain tolerance? *If yes, 3 points.* _____

   Total _____

Total of 10 to 13 points: You are *probably* endorphin-deficient.

Total of 14 or more points: You are *very probably* endorphin-deficient.

benefiting from therapy. Please note that in Appendix B, which begins on page 284, I've given some tips on how and where to purchase nutrients.

While withdrawal from opioids, including heroin, codeine, methadone, and others, can be difficult and painful, it is rarely life-threatening. If your abuse of opioids is long-term and/or severe, you are advised to consult a physician as you proceed with this program. For further information about tapering and stopping the use of these substances, see Chapter 6.

These are the primary nutrients that are often lacking in endorphin-deficient individuals:

DL-Phenylalanine (DLPA): Up to 2,000 mg, three times daily, one hour before meals. DL-phenylalanine, an amino acid, inhibits the enzyme enkephalinase, which breaks down endorphins and enkephalins at the receptor site. Please remember that if you are taking any antidepressant medication, you should consult a healthcare professional before taking phenylalanine.

L-Leucine: Up to 500 mg, three times daily, one hour before meals. The amino acid leucine is required for the production of enkephalins.

L-Methionine: Up to 500 mg, three times daily, one hour before meals. The amino acid methionine is required for the production of enkephalins.

L-Glycine: Up to 2,000 mg with each dose of DLPA. Glycine is an amino acid that helps in relaxation, and it is essential to the synthesis of endorphins and enkephalins.

L-Tyrosine: 2,000 mg, twice per day. The amino acid tyrosine is required for the production of enkephalins.

Multi-Mineral Supplement: Make sure that your mineral supplement contains the following, and take enough tablets each day to roughly equal the following dosages: calcium, 1,000 mg; magnesium, 300 mg; potassium, 100 mg; iron, 20 mg; zinc, 20 mg; manganese, 6 mg; copper, 1 mg; chromium, 400 mcg; selenium, 60 mcg; molybdenum, 50 mcg. Please note that if you are receiving dialysis treatments or have severe kidney disease, you should consult with a healthcare professional before taking any mineral supplements.

You'll want to take your Quick-Start endorphin-enkephalin supplements for at least four weeks, and probably several weeks more, depending on your results. Monitor how you feel and behave, and consult with others around you for additional input as to how you're progressing. I'm confident you'll find you're making remarkable progress during this stage of your personal Power Recovery Program.

IS YOUR SUBSTANCE PROBLEM CAUSED BY A CATECHOLAMINE DEFICIENCY?

At the age of 24, when she first came to my office, Denise L. had a ten-year history of binge eating, bulimia, mild depression, and yo-yo dieting. She began binge drinking on weekends in college. During her senior year, she began to use cocaine to give an extra "boost" to her partying. "Cocaine was it," she said. "I understood what the phrase 'drug of choice' meant the first time I used coke." She had also taken the prescription drug Ritalin on several occasions, and she told me that the way it made her feel was similar to cocaine.

"I guess I've always sort of done things in excess," she said. Denise tied her food cravings to the emotional abuse she suffered as a child. During college she had tried, for the most part successfully, to bury her boredom, emotional turmoil, and eating disorders beneath the study-hard party-hard image she cultivated.

Denise hadn't been able to "settle down" and change her behavior since she had (barely) graduated. In her words, "My best friend told me she was worried about me on several occasions, but I didn't want to listen to her and she didn't want to press it. I guess the partying finally took over. It was a way to get over the boredom, I guess. I thought, you know, that you just kind of outgrew the partying phase of your life after you got out of college, but I guess not."

Denise is a classic dopamine-deficient substance abuser, as her use of cocaine to give an extra boost to her partying and to add excitement to her life indicates. Denise's score on the catecholamine questionnaire that follows was 16, confirming that disruptions in the production of this group of neurotransmitters, of which dopamine is a member, were primary in her substance abuse problem.

Catecholamine Deficiency Questionnaire

Dopamine is produced in neurons from the amino acid tyrosine, with iron and vitamins B_3 and B_6 acting as cofactors in production. When necessary, neurons are capable of using the amino acid phenylalanine, which they convert to tyrosine, in manufacturing dopamine.

The questionnaire on page 91 will enable you to find out whether disruptions in the production of catecholamines are primary in your sub-

CATECHOLAMINE DEFICIENCY QUESTIONNAIRE

If you answer "yes" to any of the following questions, enter the number of points indicated in the blank space to the right. Enter 0 (zero) if you answer "no."

1. Is either cocaine or amphetamines your drug of choice? *If yes, 5 points.* _____

2. Do you smoke cigarettes, or use nicotine in another form, such as smokeless tobacco? *If 1 pack per day or less, 1 point. If 2 packs per day, 2 points. If 3 or more packs per day, 3 points.* _____

3. If you have used marijuana, does it excite you or have a "speedy" effect on you? *If yes, 4 points.* _____

4. Is there a history of mania in your family? *If yes, 2 points.* _____

5. Is there a history of depression in your family? *If yes, 3 points.* _____

6. Do you often experience tiredness, loss of energy, boredom, or an inability to feel pleasure? *If yes, 3 points.* _____

7. Are you a thrill-seeker or risk-taker? *If yes, 3 points.* _____

8. Do you respond positively to tricyclic antidepressant drugs, such as Tofranil, Elavil, Endep, or Pamelor? *If yes, 5 points.* _____

9. Do you respond positively to prescription drugs, such as Ritalin, Cylert, Adderall, or methamphetamine? *If yes, 5 points.* _____

10. Do antihistamine drugs like Benadryl cause you to feel "speedy?" *If yes, 2 points.* _____

    Total _____

Total of 13 to 16 points: You are *probably* catecholamine-deficient.

Total of 17 or more points: You are *very probably* catecholamine-deficient.

stance use problem. Remember, Denise's case history is just one example of the ways catecholamine deficiencies can develop and cause chemical dependencies. Even if your profile seems very different from Denise's, you should go ahead and fill in the following questionnaire. Your score will help you determine if you are catecholamine-deficient.

Essential Nutrients for Overcoming Catecholamine Deficiency

If your scores on the questionnaire on page 91 indicate that you are either *probably* or *very probably* catecholamine-deficient, disruptions in the production of catecholamines are very likely primary in your substance use problem. Listed below you will find the essential nutrients you should take to correct the nutritional deficiencies that are at the root of your catecholamine difficulty. Purchase these nutrients and begin taking them in the recommended doses as soon as possible. This should reduce or eliminate your substance urges and other symptoms within twenty-four to seventy-two hours. Please note that in Appendix B, which begins on page 285, I've given some tips on how and where to purchase nutrients.

These are the core nutrients that are often undersupplied in catecholamine-deficient individuals:

L-Tyrosine: Up to 1,500 mg, three times daily, one hour before meals. Tyrosine, an amino acid, is the primary nutrient required by neurons to produce catecholamines. In cases of severe cocaine, Ritalin, or amphetamine abuse, as many as 2,500 mg of tyrosine can be taken, three times per day. Please note that tyrosine is a safe and natural amino acid supplement, but it can have a stimulating effect. If you are taking antidepressant medication, you should consult with a healthcare professional before taking tyrosine. This stimulation may, in rare cases, cause a mild increase in blood pressure. If you have a history of hypertension, regular blood pressure checks are recommended. In addition, if you have a history of melanoma, you should not take tyrosine.

L-Glutamine: Up to 1,000 mg, three times daily, one hour before meals. Glutamine is an amino acid that helps in relaxation and helps to stabilize blood sugar levels. It is available in tablet and powder form. (The powder is less expensive). Please note that if you have cirrhosis of the liver or severe liver disease, you should consult with a healthcare professional before taking glutamine.

B-Complex Vitamin Capsule, or Multi-Vitamin with High Levels of B Vitamins: At least one capsule, three times daily, with tyrosine and glutamine. Vitamin B_3 (niacin), folic acid, vitamin B_6 (pyridoxine), vitamin C, iron, and copper are all required for the production of catecholamines. Your B-vitamin tablet should contain at least 50 mg of vitamins B_3 and B_6, but you should take less than 300 mg per day of each.

To avoid "niacin flush," an unpleasant reddening and sensitivity of the skin from too much niacin, make sure the niacin in your B-vitamin supplement is in the form of niacinamide or inositol hexaniacinate. Your B-vitamin capsule should also contain at least 400 mcg of folic acid, and it's okay to take up to 1,000 mcg, or 1 mg, of this vitamin. Please note that taking a B-vitamin supplement may make your urine bright yellow. This is perfectly normal and is a result of your body's elimination of B vitamins which it can't use.

Vitamin C: At least 500 mg, three times daily. Vitamin C is another important cofactor in the production of catecholamines, and up to 5,000 mg per day can safely be taken. Please note that large doses of vitamin C may cause loose bowel movements. If this occurs, reduce your vitamin C dosage until you resume normal bowel movements.

Multi-Mineral Supplement: The minerals you need may be included in a multi-vitamin, multi-mineral supplement. If you choose to take a separate mineral supplement, make sure it contains the following, and take enough tablets each day to roughly equal the following dosages: calcium, 1,000 mg; magnesium, 300 mg; potassium, 100 mg; iron, 20 mg; zinc, 20 mg; manganese, 6 mg; copper, 1 mg; chromium, 400 mcg; selenium, 60 mcg; molybdenum, 50 mcg. Please note that if you are receiving dialysis treatments or have severe kidney disease, you should consult with a healthcare professional before taking mineral supplements.

You'll want to take your Quick-Start catecholamine supplements for at least four weeks, and probably several weeks more, depending on your results. Monitor how you feel and behave, and consult with others around you for additional input as to how you're progressing. I'm confident you'll find you're making remarkable progress during this stage of your personal Power Recovery Program.

QUICK-START FOR SMOKERS

If you've identified a problem with one or more neurotransmitters in the previous four questionnaires, skip this section. Simply add the nutrient lecithin from the list below, but do not add the other nutritional supplements, even if you are a smoker. You'll likely find that the nutrients you're taking for your other neurotransmitter deficiency or deficiencies will also help reduce your urge for nicotine.

If smoking or using smokeless tobacco is your only substance problem, this section is for you. I've included this special Quick-Start for Smokers section because nicotine, the psychotropic substance in tobacco, is very different from most other substances. While almost all of the other substances I deal with in this book achieve their effects by disrupting one primary neurotransmitter, nicotine acts on several.

Nicotine achieves its initial effects by disrupting the neurotransmitter acetylcholine. Like other neurotransmitters, acetylcholine has several different subtypes of receptor with which it can combine. One group, called nicotinic receptors, can also be occupied by nicotine molecules. Unlike those of most other substances, however, nicotine's effects quickly spread to each of the four major neurotransmitters I've discussed. In other words, nicotine also disrupts serotonin, endorphins and enkephalins, dopamine, and GABA. To complicate matters further, nicotine's effects can vary dramatically from one person to the next. Many people use tobacco because it helps them concentrate and stay alert, while others use it to relax. Because it stimulates both inhibitory and excitatory neurotransmitters, nicotine is capable of both energizing and relaxing.

Nicotine provides a perfect example of the individuality of our "biochemical fingerprints." Nicotine's effects on tobacco users depend partly on which of the secondary neurotransmitters in the brain are the most strongly stimulated by the substance. That's why I recommend that if you use other substances besides tobacco, you answer the Quick-Start questionnaires and take the nutrients to replenish your primary neurotransmitter shortage. Many people find that taking the Quick-Start nutrients to replenish one or two primary neurotransmitters and reduce drug and alcohol cravings also reduces their urge to smoke at the same time.

Essential Nutrients for Overcoming Nicotine Addiction

These are the primary nutrients that will help replenish the neurotransmitters disrupted by nicotine. Taking these nutrients should address your core nutrient shortages and reduce or eliminate your cigarette or smokeless tobacco cravings in a short time.

Purified Lecithin: Up to 2,000 mg, three times daily, one hour before breakfast and dinner, and at bedtime. Our bodies are able to use the choline derived from this nutritional supplement to boost the production of the neurotransmitter acetylcholine and counteract the effects of nicotine, which directly disrupts the production of acetylcholine. Please note that if you suffer from Parkinson's Disease, you should consult a healthcare professional before taking lecithin.

L-Tyrosine: Up to 2,000 mg, three times daily, one hour before meals. Tyrosine, an amino acid, is the primary nutrient required by neurons to produce catecholamines, whose production is indirectly disrupted by the use of nicotine. Please note that if you are taking antidepressant medication, you should consult a healthcare professional before taking tyrosine.

5HTP: Up to 200 mg, three times daily, one hour before breakfast and dinner, and at bedtime. 5HTP, which is synthesized as part of the serotonin production process in the brain, is the primary nutrient required by neurons to produce serotonin. Serotonin is another neurotransmitter indirectly affected by nicotine.

Tryptophan, an amino acid, is the primary nutrient required by neurons to produce serotonin, and it can be used in place of 5HTP. 5HTP is made from tryptophan during the serotonin production cycle, and 5HTP is about ten times stronger than tryptophan, so it will help you restore your serotonin levels more quickly than tryptophan. Some people, however, respond better to tryptophan than to 5HTP, although the reasons for this are unknown. If you take tryptophan, you should take 1,000 to 2,000 mg, three times per day. Tryptophan and 5HTP can be taken together. Please note that if you are taking antidepressant medication, you should consult with a healthcare professional before taking 5HTP or tryptophan.

L-Glutamine: Up to 1,000 mg, three times daily, one hour before meals. Glutamine is an amino acid that helps in relaxation. It is available in tablet and powder form. (The powder is less expensive). Please note that if you have cirrhosis of the liver or severe liver disease, you should consult with a healthcare professional before taking glutamine.

B-Complex Vitamin Capsule: At least one capsule, twice daily, with phenylalanine. Several B vitamins, including vitamin B_3 (niacin), folic acid, vitamin B_5 (pantothenic acid), and vitamin B_6 (pyridoxine), are important cofactors in the production of these important neurotransmitters.

To avoid "niacin flush," an unpleasant reddening and sensitivity of the skin from too much niacin, make sure the niacin in your B-vitamin supplement is in the form of niacinamide or inositol hexaniacinate. Note that taking a B-vitamin supplement may make your urine bright yellow. This is perfectly normal and is a result of your body's elimination of B vitamins which it can't use.

Vitamin C: At least 1,500 mg, three times daily. Please note that smokers may need as much as 10,000 mg of vitamin C daily as an antioxidant to help counteract the effects of smoking.

Multi-Mineral Supplement: The minerals you need may be included in a multi-vitamin, multi-mineral supplement. If you choose to take a separate mineral supplement, make sure it contains the following, and take enough tablets each day to roughly equal the following dosages: calcium, 1,000 mg; magnesium, 300 mg; potassium, 100 mg; iron, 20 mg; zinc, 20 mg; manganese, 6 mg; copper, 1 mg; chromium, 400 mcg; selenium, 60 mcg; molybdenum, 50 mcg. Please note that if you use nicotine to relax, you will want to take 20 to 25 mg of additional zinc each day. If you use nicotine to improve your focus and energy levels, you'll want to make sure that your supplements contain copper and that you take at least 2 mg of copper per day.

It is also important to note that if you are receiving dialysis treatments or have severe kidney disease, you should consult with a healthcare professional before taking mineral supplements. And if you smoke less than a pack of cigarettes per day, you need to take the Quick-Start for Smokers nutrients only twice per day.

Possible Side Effects of the Quick-Start for Smokers Nutrients

While I've mentioned a few things, such as bright yellow urine caused by B vitamins, which you might notice as you take your Quick-Start supplements, nicotine users, especially those who use nicotine patches or nicotine gum, may experience other symptoms. Let me talk briefly about a few of them here.

Many people who use the Quick-Start for Smokers nutrients find that they become very lethargic within a day or two of starting the nutrients. This is because the Quick-Start nutrients are working! The nutrients are actually enabling the brain to increase the production of the neurotransmitters disrupted by nicotine, causing the effect of the nicotine to be magnified. If you experience this side effect, cut back on the amount of nicotine you're using or discontinue the use of nicotine altogether. You should quickly regain your normal energy levels. You'll be surprised at how little nicotine you really need if your brain is given what it needs to function normally.

The symptoms of queasiness and/or lightheadedness are, again, an indicator that the Quick-Start for Smokers nutrients are working. What you're really experiencing are the toxic effects of nicotine. These symptoms may be very similar to what you felt when you smoked your first cigarettes. They're a dramatic indicator of how toxic a substance nicotine is. Again, if you experience these side effects, cut back on your nicotine intake or discontinue the use of nicotine altogether. Your symptoms should disappear very quickly.

You'll want to take your Quick-Start for Smokers supplements for at least four weeks, and probably several weeks more, depending on your results. Monitor how you feel and behave, and consult with others around you for additional input as to how you're progressing. I'm confident you'll find you're making remarkable progress during this stage of your personal Power Recovery Program.

QUICK-START FOR MARIJUANA USERS

If you've identified a problem with one or more neurotransmitters in the previous four questionnaires, skip this section. Simply add the nutrient lecithin from the list below, but do not add the other nutritional supplements, even if you are a marijuana user. You'll likely find that the nutrients you're taking for your other neurotransmitter deficiency or deficiencies will also help reduce your urge for marijuana. In addition to adding the lecithin from the list below, you can also purchase "granular lecithin" and add it to soups, salads, and other foods.

If marijuana use or abuse is your only substance problem, this section is for you. I've included the Quick-Start for Marijuana Users section because THC (tetrahydrocannabinol), one the main psychotropic substances in marijuana, is very different from most other psychoactive substances. This difference lies in the fact that the brain's natural cannabinoids (the neurotransmitter anandamide is the best understood of these) work in reverse from the way other neurotransmitters work. Anandamide functions by damping down the effects of other neurotransmitters as it moves from a receiving neuron to a sending neuron, precisely backwards from the normal neurotransmitter process. This process is called "retrograde signaling." This causes inhibitory feedback on the cell releasing other neurotransmitters and damps down their effects. Many marijuana abusers will state that one of the effects of marijuana is that it allows them to "chill out," which is exactly what the purpose of the brain's natural endocannabinoids is.

Natural endocannabinoids achieve their effects by stimulating cannabinoid receptors on cells that release neurotransmitters like GABA and dopamine, thus downregulating them. Endocannabinoids are made from arachidonic acid, a constituent in animal fat and butter and various components in lecithin, a type of fat that is concentrated in organ meats like liver, in legumes such as beans, and in eggs. The dangerous low-fat, low-cholesterol diet craze and the disappearance of these dense high-fat and high-protein foods from the modern diet deprive the brain of the precursor molecules which are required to synthesize the natural endocannabinoids, so the increasing popularity of marijuana is easy to understand.

Because lecithin is an important precursor for the brain's production of acetylcholine ("natural nicotine") and anandamide ("natural cannabinoid"), most teenagers who smoke marijuana also smoke cigarettes. The emphasis on diets which are deficient in organ meats, eggs, and legumes, which are natural sources of this nutrient, certainly goes a long way to explain this.

Listed below are the primary nutrients that will help replenish the natural cannabinoid neurotransmitters disrupted by the artificial cannabinoids in marijuana. Taking these nutrients should address your core nutrient shortages and reduce or eliminate your marijuana cravings in a short time. Please note that in Appendix B, which begins on page 284, I've given some tips on how and where to purchase nutrients.

Purified Lecithin: Up to 2,000 mg, three times daily, with meals. Our bodies are able to process certain phospholipids in lecithin, such as phosphatidyl choline and phosphatidyl ethanolamine, to boost the production of the neurotransmitter endocannabinoids such as anadamide, which counteracts the effects of the artificial disruption of cannabinoids caused by using marijuana and hashish. Also, you can add several teaspoonfuls of "granular lecithin" to soups, salad dressings, and other foods to get extra phospholipids. Adding extra eggs, legumes, and organ meats such as liver to the diet can help also. Please note that if you suffer from Parkinson's Disease, you should consult a healthcare professional before taking phosphatidyl choline.

Organic Butter and Animal Fats: One of the components of animal fat is arachidonic acid, which is also needed to synthesize endocannabinoids, and although it can be obtained from lecithin and phospholipids-rich foods such as eggs and organ meats, organic butter is a rich source of arachidonic acid and other essential nutrients. I recommend that you consume organic butter liberally.

Vitamin E: Up to 800 IU per day. The four kinds of vitamin E (called tocopherols) and the closely related tocotrienols have antioxidant benefits for fatty tissues and molecules such as those which make up cell membranes. Cannabinoids are fat-soluble molecules, which is why they can linger in the body for long periods of time, and they ultimately need to be oxidized and cleared. This detoxification process can be assisted by vitamin E.

Muti-Vitamin/Multi-Mineral Capsule: At least one capsule, twice daily, for basic nutrition. Please note that for marijuana users who are over 35 years old, the high-animal-fat diet suggested above should be balanced with extra fish oils, either through taking them as supplements or consuming fish such as salmon, mackerel, herring, or trout, to counteract the diet's potentially artery-damaging effects.

You'll want to take your Quick-Start for Marijuana Users supplements for at least four weeks, and probably several weeks more, depending on your results. Monitor how you feel and behave, and consult with others around you for additional input as to how you're progressing. I'm confident you'll find you're making remarkable progress during this stage of your personal Power Recovery Program.

THE COST OF NUTRITIONAL SUPPLEMENTS

Many of my patients ask me how much it's going to cost them to buy their Power Recovery Program nutrients. The most accurate answer I can give to this question is, "They're free." Of course, I don't mean that you won't have to buy them. What I mean is that you should add up the dollar cost of the substance or substances you won't be buying, and compare that to what you'll be paying for nutrients. More than 75 percent of my patients who did that calculation agreed with me: "They're free." And most of my past patients who quit smoking through my program were paying a lot less than the $7.00 per pack of cigarettes many people pay today. Of course, marijuana users pay much more to support their addictions.

In practical terms, the cost of Quick-Start nutrients will vary depending on which nutrients you're using, the brand of nutrients you buy, and where you buy them. But most people report that the Quick-Start nutrients cost from $3.00 to $6.00 per day, less than an inexpensive lunch. If you'd like to present your nutritional supplement bills to your health insurance provider, you can ask your physician to write a letter stating that the Power Recovery Program nutrients are medically necessary. In some cases, health insurance may cover their costs, but in general most insurance plans will not pay for products that are available without a prescription. The cost of nutritional supplements is a tax deductible medical expense if a physician has recommended them.

TAKING THE QUICK-START SUPPLEMENTS

Let me emphasize again that all of the nutrients I recommend in the

Power Recovery Program are completely natural, non-toxic substances. In fact, they're in many of the foods you eat every day, although for various reasons you may not be able to utilize them in producing several key neurotransmitters. As you progress with the Quick-Start stage, you'll be building up your body's reserves of the nutrients you're taking, so you may find that you can begin to gradually reduce the amounts of your Quick-Start nutrients in as few as four to six weeks. Generally speaking, however, I recommend that you take the Quick-Start nutrients for three to six months before beginning to taper off their use.

Before you purchase your Quick-Start supplements and begin taking them, I'd like give to you an idea of what you can expect, based on what my patients have reported to me. After you've been taking your Quick-Start nutrients for two or three days, most of you will notice positive changes in the way you feel. You may find that you're more focused, or that your energy level has increased, or that some of the little things that typically bother you don't seem quite as irritating as they did. You may discover that your sleep patterns have improved and that your outlook has brightened noticeably. For many of you, once your Quick-Start nutrients begin to take effect, the sheer *physical* urge to use drugs or alcohol will simply not be as powerful as it has been. Perhaps your reduction in cravings will be subtle; perhaps it will be quite dramatic.

But even if you don't think you notice changes, be careful of concluding that the Quick-Start nutrients aren't having a positive effect. Frequently my patients will state that the Quick-Start nutrients failed to work, only to be contradicted by a friend or family member who had noticed marked improvements in the patient's moods and behavior. Other people often have a more objective view of how we act than we ourselves do, so before deciding that Quick-Start is not working, you might want to get some feedback from those close to you. You might also want to take an objective look at your own behavior. Are you spending more time with your family? Are you getting caught up on odd jobs around the house that you've neglected for a long time? Have others remarked that you seem to have more energy? Many of my patients have found that Quick-Start was working even before they realized it.

I want to talk about another important topic: continued substance use. During the Quick-Start stage, most people find that, as their irritability, anxiety, and mood swings diminish and they regain the ability to concentrate, their need to use substances is also significantly reduced. As a result, they often begin to reduce their substance use or stop completely within the first few days. But let me emphasize one thing: Don't worry if you continue your substance use during the first few days of the Quick-Start stage. Remember, you're just beginning to get your disrupted neurotransmitter production back to normal, and how quickly that is accomplished depends upon how serious the disruption is. On the other hand, as your need to use your substance diminishes, I certainly recommend that you also reduce or stop your substance use during these first days. If you're going to AA meetings or using prayer or meditation or psychotherapy to help in your recovery, remember that your ability to benefit from these therapies will improve enormously as you rebalance your brain chemistry. I'll talk in more detail about stopping substance use completely in the next chapter on Stage Two, Detoxification.

In some cases, however, the Quick-Start nutrients don't bring about positive mood changes and reductions in cravings. There are various reasons for this, the most common of which is that your system is highly toxic. In other words, stress, toxin exposure, and/or drug use have caused a heavy buildup of toxins in your body and your brain, and these toxins are preventing you from absorbing, utilizing, and realizing the benefits of the Quick-Start nutrients. As you begin taking the nutrients for Stage Two, Detoxification, you will be better able to fully take advantage of Quick-Start.

Remember that after you've been taking your Quick-Start nutrients for a short time—from two or three days to two weeks—I want to encourage you to add the Detoxification nutrients to your regimen. Many people find that they need to take both the Quick-Start and Detoxification nutrients together for anywhere from eight weeks to as many as seven or eight months to fully restore their neurotransmitter balance. After that, many of my patients taper their dosages of these nutrients. This means that they may take them only once per day instead of two or three times per day. Many find that they can reduce their Quick-Start nutrients to three or four times per week. You can be the judge of when to taper these dosages, but don't be surprised if your need for them is still there for three months or more. The important thing is that your symptoms associated with substance use will very likely be reduced or even eliminated, and that's one of the first steps to successful recovery.

In Appendix B (see page 284) you'll find a list of recommended resources for the purchase of nutritional supplements and for finding support for your recovery. I've also included several nutritional supplement checklists in Appendix A (see page 275) to help you keep daily track of the supplements you take.

CONCLUSION

Remember that, just as no two people are alike, no two people have exactly the same response to drugs and alcohol. Everyone reacts in different ways to different drugs, depending on his genetic and biochemical make-up, nutritional health, and toxic load. The Power Recovery Program will enable you to tailor a recovery strategy to your biochemical needs. You're taking the first important step with the Quick-Start stage. By the time you've completed all three stages of the Power Recovery Program, you'll have developed a personal regimen of nutritional supplements to help you maintain the biochemical balance you need to be healthy and substance-free, like thousands of others who have used my program.

6

Stage Two
Detoxification

You've begun the Quick-Start stage of the Power Recovery Program, and you're taking nutritional supplements designed to quickly raise the blood levels of specific nutrients which will give your brain the necessary "building blocks" to resume normal production of the key neurotransmitters your substance use has disrupted. Now you're ready to begin Stage 2, Detoxification.

Ideally, you should begin this stage within two or three days to a week after you begin taking your Quick-Start nutrients, although you can wait for as long as two weeks to start. Many of my patients find they're more comfortable letting their bodies "get used to the Quick-Start nutrients" for a few weeks before they begin Detoxification. As I said in the Introduction to Part II, you'll be taking both your Quick-Start and Detoxification nutrients together. The sooner you begin the Detoxification stage, the sooner you'll be able to eliminate one of the other primary stumbling blocks in the recovery process. In this chapter I'll show you how to use nutritional supplements to help cleanse your body of the toxins that may be preventing you from absorbing the Quick-Start nutrients and reestablishing normal neurotransmitter production.

Let me add an important qualifier here: The Detoxification stage of the Power Recovery Program is not just for people with substance problems. It can also provide great benefits even to those who are not substance users. Almost everyone has a need to help her body process and eliminate toxins, and my detoxification protocol is a safe and natural way to do that.

RESPONDING TO THE POWER RECOVERY PROGRAM THUS FAR

Most of you who have begun taking your Quick-Start nutrients will already have noticed positive changes in the way you feel. For many of you, these changes might include a significant reduction in your need to use drugs or alcohol. Some of you will find your substance cravings have disappeared. You may also notice that your moods have improved, you're able to concentrate better, and your sleep disturbances are not as bad as they were. In some cases, however, these Quick-Start benefits might not have kicked in yet. The degree to which the Quick-Start nutrients reduce your cravings and improve the way you feel and function depends on a number of factors. Primary among these is the degree of toxicity of your body. To put it another way, toxicity refers to the level (or "load") of toxins which your body must eliminate. If you have a high toxic load, your body may have difficulty absorbing and using your Quick-Start nutrients, and you may not yet be feeling the positive changes I've talked about.

Although thousands of my patients have realized immediate benefits from their Quick-Start nutrients, I've also treated some for whom Quick-Start didn't work as expected. In most of these cases, however, they were able to experience the positive results that the Quick-Start nutrients can bring about within a matter of four to six weeks *after* they began the Detoxification stage of the Power Recovery Program. If you experience this type of delay, don't give up. Be sure to continue taking your Quick-Start nutrients along with your Detoxification nutrients as you progress through this next stage.

For those of you who have noticed reductions in your substance cravings and improvements in the way you feel and function, imagine those positive changes magnified several times and you'll have an idea of what's ahead. Now let's get started with Stage Two of the Power Recovery Program: Detoxification. And remember, I invite all of you, even those who do not have substance problems, to take the Detoxification nutrients.

DEFINING DETOXIFICATION

If you've ever been a patient at a drug and alcohol recovery facility, or if you've talked with someone who has, you've got an idea of how most professionals who treat substance problems define detoxification. For them, detoxification refers to a period of time (usually several days at most) during which most of an abused substance is processed and excreted from a patient's body. The key to achieving this is abstinence from the substance. After enough time has elapsed for a patient's body to have gotten rid of most detectable residues of the substance of abuse, she is considered "detoxified." In other words, the only toxins most addictions professionals deal with are the specific substances for which their patients are being treated.

From what you now know about the risk factors for substance problems and about why symptoms related to substance use occur, it will be clear to you that this definition of detoxification falls woefully short of the mark. Traces of substances of abuse and the byproducts of these substances which occur as the body metabolizes them can remain in the body for long periods of time, from several months to years. Environmental toxins and other toxins related to substance use (cadmium, from smoking, for example) can remain in the body, further interfere with normal biochemistry, and diminish the likelihood of a successful recovery. To further complicate matters, many addictions professionals routinely prescribe other psychotropic toxins, including tranquilizers, antidepressants, and *substitute* drugs, during what they call detoxification. As you've seen, these substances add to the toxic load the body must deal with. They often make things worse, not better, and, except in cases (which I'll discuss) where withdrawal symptoms can be life-threatening, they are usually not necessary for detoxification.

My own definition of the term *detoxification* is much broader and more inclusive. First, let me repeat the obvious: There are often many different toxins involved in causing the biochemical imbalances that are at the root of substance cravings. Based on this, *detoxification* means to me *the removal of any toxic substances, both psychotropic and non-psychotropic, that have accumulated in your body.*

As I've pointed out previously, these toxic substances may be residues from your cigarette, drug, or alcohol use, or dietary and environmental toxins you've been exposed to, or toxins resulting from the overgrowth of harmful intestinal flora, especially yeast. No matter what their origin, it is important to interrupt the source of toxins during this stage of the Power Recovery Program. If you have a high toxic load, you may have difficulty reducing or eliminating your substance use, simply because you may be using drugs and alcohol to mask symptoms caused by poisons that have accumulated in your body. In addition, a high toxic load may put you at risk for developing harmful degenerative conditions in the future. As I've said, it's very likely that many of the toxins which are disrupting your brain chemistry have been accumulating since before you started using cigarettes, drugs, or alcohol. By taking steps to remove them, along with residues of your substance of abuse, you'll be significantly improving the way you feel and function, and enhancing your chances to remain substance-free.

WHY WE NEED THE DETOXIFICATION STAGE

The Detoxification stage of the Power Recovery Program is the second and final key step for most problem substance users. Especially if you have a relatively short history of substance abuse, as most users do, you'll find that combining this stage with Quick-Start will enable you to reduce your symptoms and eliminate toxins that are very likely causing those symptoms, often virtually eliminating the likelihood of your relapsing into substance use.

With this in mind, the goals of the Detoxification stage of the Power Recovery Program are:

• Removing the sources of toxins that can poison your brain and body and which can contribute to the nutritional deficiencies and biochemical imbalances that have put you at risk for substance problems.

• Fortifying the "toxin barriers" of your digestive system so that toxins you ingest are not readily absorbed.

• Strengthening your body's detoxification pathways so that the ongoing process of detoxification can be carried out with maximum efficiency.

The Detoxification stage of the Power Recovery Program consists of a protocol of nine nutritional supplements which are specifically designed to detoxify your body and enable you to achieve the three goals I've listed above. I want to make it clear from the outset that, in most cases, these are not goals that can be accomplished overnight. The process of getting rid of accumulated toxins is necessarily a gradual one, and it generally takes longer than reversing nutritional deficiencies. But while it may take some time for you to eliminate most of your toxic load, the good news is that most of you will *begin* to feel the positive results of your Power Recovery Program detoxification within a short time, in some cases only a few weeks. If your toxic load is high, and your body's ability to detoxify seriously impaired, the process may take several months.

STOPPING SUBSTANCE USE

Now I've got to introduce a word into this discussion that many people who have substance problems dread hearing. The word is *withdrawal.* Withdrawal symptoms are part of the detoxification process, and almost everyone who has a substance problem experiences them to some degree as she cuts down on or stops substance use and begins to detoxify. For many of you, the Quick-Start nutrients will have such a pronounced positive effect that you might not even be aware that you're in withdrawal. Others might notice withdrawal symptoms but find that, because of the beneficial effects of the Quick-Start nutrients, they're not really too bad.

But it's important to remember that withdrawal is a very real and sometimes dangerous phase of recovery from a substance use problem. I want to discuss it at some length here, because under certain conditions withdrawal can be life-threatening. It's not something to be taken lightly. I also want to make it clear that it is absolutely safe to take the Power Recovery Program Quick-Start and Detoxification nutrients as you taper and eventually stop your substance use. While, as I've said, in some cases withdrawal from substance use can be difficult or dangerous, taking nutritional supplements during withdrawal will not put you in any danger and will probably improve your outcome significantly. With that in mind, here are some guidelines to help you decide whether you can safely discontinue your substance use without medical help during detoxification or whether you need to seek professional supervision during withdrawal.

Let me start by suggesting that you ask yourself a few questions about your substance use. First, are you at risk for developing a biochemical dependence on your substance of abuse? For those of you who use alcohol, if you've been averaging more than four drinks per day, even for only a few weeks, you're at risk for dependence, and therefore for withdrawal symptoms. Smoking a pack or more of cigarettes per day for longer than a few months also puts you at risk. And with stimulants such as cocaine or amphetamine substances, you may be at risk for dependence after as few as three to four weeks of taking these substances an average of four times per week or more. With serotonin-selective reuptake inhibitors (SSRIs), dependence can develop in two to three months, while with the benzodiazepine family of prescription psychotropic drugs, dependence can develop in as little as five to seven days.

Next, how serious is your substance use problem? Let me give you some questions which will help you determine this. Have you in the past ever quit using your substance of abuse abruptly after an extended period of steady use? If so, what withdrawal symptoms did you experience? If, for instance, you use alcohol regularly and consume an average of four or more drinks per day, but periodically stop drinking for several days or longer, are your withdrawal symptoms something you can live with? Perhaps you experience headaches, listlessness, and a mild case of the "shakes" for a few days, but then you begin to get back to normal. In cases such as this, where you've experienced withdrawal in the past and found your symptoms manageable, you are not likely to have serious problems tapering or discontinuing your drinking during detoxification, especially with the help of the Quick-Start and Detoxification nutrients.

If you're a cocaine user, do you use the drug every day, or are there periods of several days or more between the times you use the drug? Are you able to deal with the letdown you experience during cocaine withdrawal? If so, you should not have a problem when you stop using cocaine during detoxification. In fact, although "coming down" from a cocaine "high" can be emotionally draining, withdrawing from cocaine rarely causes life-threatening physical symptoms. By the same token, while withdrawal from opiates (including heroin, morphine, codeine, methadone, and prescription painkillers) is often accompanied by nausea, physical discomfort, and severe cravings, it too is rarely life-threatening.

There's one final thing you should note. If you're over 60 years of age or are suffering from other medical or psychiatric problems which can lower your tolerance of physical or emotional stress such as that which might occur during withdrawal from substance use, you should strongly consider getting professional medical help during this period.

In general, the guidelines that I had set for you are as follows. If you have gradually reduced your substance use, or you have stopped it altogether in the past and have been able to easily cope with withdrawal symptoms, you should have no problem quitting during your Power Recover Program Detoxification. If you are a cigarette smoker, a casual drinker, or an occasional drug user who is attempting to quit because you're beginning to notice the negative effects of your substance use, you too can almost certainly stop your substance use as you proceed with the Detoxification stage.

There are, however, several instances where you must proceed very cautiously when considering how to discontinue substance use during a detoxification process. Let me give you some examples. In cases of severe alcoholism, withdrawal can be life-threatening. Alcohol detoxification has been broken down into well-defined stages, each of which is characterized by the severity of the withdrawal symptoms. One of the most dangerous, Delirium Tremens, or the DTs, can end in death if it is not properly and closely supervised. *If you are at risk for the serious, life-threatening withdrawal symptoms associated with advanced alcoholism, you should not attempt to taper or discontinue alcohol use outside of a professional addictions treatment facility.*

If you are taking any of the benzodiazepines, such as Valium, Klonopin, Ativan, or Xanax, you may also experience serious, potentially life-threatening withdrawal symptoms. If you suddenly stop taking these drugs or taper their use too rapidly, you put yourself at risk for physically painful, emotionally wrenching symptoms, and for seizures which can result in death. *Do not attempt to rapidly taper or completely discontinue the use of these substances without professional supervision. Admission to a substance recovery and detoxification facility may be necessary during withdrawal from these substances.*

The onset of the mood-altering effects of serotonin-selective reuptake inhibitors (SSRIs) is more gradual than those of drugs which disrupt the normal GABA cycle, and withdrawal symptoms associated with stopping the use of SSRIs likewise tend to manifest more gradually and be less severe than those of the benzodiazepines. The most common symptoms of SSRI withdrawal include extreme irritability and anxious depression, which can trigger a strong desire to begin taking SSRIs again. These symptoms can continue until your brain chemistry begins to be rebalanced and the normal production, release, and reuptake of serotonin are reestablished. *Because of the risk of serious rebound depression, you should be*

monitored by your physician or an addictions treatment professional as you taper
the use of an SSRI or any other prescription psychotropic substance.

If you've ever had a withdrawal experience which required medical
intervention, you should consult a physician or an addictions treatment
professional before you abruptly stop your substance use. Finally, even if
your answers to the questions above indicate that you're probably not at
risk if you stop your substance use, *if you have any doubts about whether you*
should quit your substance use abruptly, consult a healthcare professional or a
professional in the field of addictions treatment.

Likewise, if you're using a substance I have not covered in the preced-
ing discussion, and you're not sure about the effects of suddenly stopping
its use, consult your physician or an addictions treatment specialist. In
any case, whether you choose to taper off or stop your substance use on
your own or under professional supervision, the combination of Quick-
Start and Detoxification nutrients can safely assist you in any withdrawal
process.

WHAT TO EXPECT DURING WITHDRAWAL

Although each type of psychotropic substance has characteristic withdrawal symptoms, no two people have exactly the same withdrawal
experience. Your drug or alcohol use has caused disruptions in neurotransmitter production, and your brain has responded by trying to
reestablish biochemical balance in the presence of the substance. For most
drugs, this means that the brain has *down-regulated* (or reduced) the number of receptors for a particular neurotransmitter, or has lessened its production of the neurotransmitter itself, although there are some drugs
which cause the brain to overproduce neurotransmitters or *up-regulate*
receptors to compensate for their effects.

When you discontinue the use of drugs or alcohol, the abnormal biochemical balances that were achieved artificially to compensate for the
effects of the abused substance become once again unbalanced. Your system is, in effect, shocked into trying to establish a new biochemical balance which does not depend on an external psychotropic substance. The
Quick-Start nutrients are targeted at quickly providing your brain the necessary "building blocks" to begin producing neurotransmitters at a normal level and thus reduce the effects of withdrawal.

Even so, withdrawal from virtually any psychotropic substance is usually accompanied by irritability, tiredness or listlessness, and lack of focus. If you've been using a substance for a relatively short time, your symptoms might be mild. For instance, most people who use drugs on a regular but intermittent basis and are in good health find that because of the positive effects of the Quick-Start nutrients, alcohol and/or drug detoxification usually entails no more than a day or two of irritability and mild cravings. For some people, withdrawal is also accompanied by headaches and sleep disturbances. If your substance use is such that you're not at risk for serious withdrawal symptoms, you should be able to stop without too much discomfort.

Remember, restoring the nutrients needed for normal neuron function is the only way to rebalance brain chemistry disrupted by substance abuse. The suggestion that the use of other drugs, including prescription drugs, can restore normal brain function is simply not true. In fact, using other psychotropic substances can only make brain chemistry more unbalanced than it has been and will significantly delay recovery.

The Power Recovery Program Quick-Start and Detoxification nutrients will, in most cases, enable you to function more normally in your daily life while you taper off and discontinue substance use. Many of you will find, in fact, that you're actually coping better *without* your substance of choice because you're beginning to naturally restore the production of the neurotransmitters which will truly help you deal with stress.

WHAT CAUSES TOXIC LOAD
AND HOW DOES THE BODY DEAL WITH IT?

I've talked at some length about what toxic load is and why it's important to remove toxins from your body. Now I'd like to spend some time discussing how it happens and what some of its consequences are. There are three main causes of high toxic load.

The first main cause is *high exposure to toxins.* Our bodies make extensive use of molecules of the mineral sulfur to combine with numerous toxic substances, including some heavy metals, in order to prepare them for elimination. This process is called *chelation* (kee-LAY-shun). Chelation is one of the natural processes our bodies employ as part of detoxification. When our bodies have too great a toxic load, we use up sulfur-containing nutrients as we try to chelate out the toxins. This can result in a shortage of sulfur nutrients, impairing our ability to perform this important function.

The second main cause of high toxic load is *breakdowns of the body's barriers against toxins*. The barriers which are critical in preventing toxins from entering our blood and lymph systems include the following:

• Stomach acid, which kills many potentially harmful bacteria and parasites in the food and water we consume.

• Digestive enzymes in the stomach and small intestines, which break down food into nutrient molecules that can be used by our cells.

• Beneficial intestinal flora, which compete with harmful bacteria, yeast, and parasites to maintain a healthy intestinal balance.

• The intestinal wall, which normally screens out toxins while allowing nutrient molecules to pass through to the blood and lymph.

• The immune system, which responds to foreign substances, including toxins and microorganisms which manage to pass through the first four barriers.

• The liver, which filters and removes toxins from nutrient-rich blood after it leaves the intestines.

When these barriers are intact, our natural ability to process and eliminate toxic substances usually enables us to live healthy lives. When one or more of them break down, we're likely to suffer from excessive toxic load.

Finally, the third main cause of high toxic load is *the inability of the liver to adequately process toxins*. The liver is, in a sense, the final barrier to toxins, because it is in the liver that a final toxin removal takes place before digested molecules absorbed from the intestine make their way into the bloodstream. Under normal circumstances, even when toxins have managed to enter the bloodstream from some source other than the digestive tract, they must pass through the liver, where they undergo a two-step removal process. First, toxins are turned into *free radicals*, molecules which are ready to combine with other substances to prepare them for removal from the body. Although free radicals can be very damaging (they're often more dangerous than the toxins they're made from), in the controlled environment of the liver, the free radical stage is required to prepare toxins for the next step in removal.

Next, these free radical toxins are *conjugated*. This means that they combine with one of four other types of molecule—glycine, glutathione, glucuronide, or sulfur—in the liver. Conjugated toxin molecules are then eliminated through the urine or the stool.

It is usually through high toxin exposure or the breakdown of one or more of these critical conjugation pathways in our bodies that high toxic load occurs, and this is common among substance users. The important thing, though, is that in most cases excess toxicity is a correctable condition. The Power Recovery Program Detoxification nutrients which I'll prescribe are specifically designed to counteract these breakdowns and eliminate excess toxic load. Adding them to your Quick-Start nutrients can enable most of you to complete your return to substance-free good health by restoring your body's ability to eliminate toxins.

In addition to contributing to substance cravings, high toxic load can cause other symptoms, including headaches, memory loss, intestinal problems, and mood disorders. I've found that a significant percentage of the patients I treat for substance use problems also have other symptoms related to toxicity, and, in fact, they might have begun their substance use in the first place to help deal with symptoms caused by high levels of toxins in their bodies. In Chapter 17, I've included case histories to illustrate the kinds of symptoms that can result from each of the three primary causes of high toxic load.

NUTRITIONAL SUPPLEMENTS THAT WILL HELP YOU WIN THE BATTLE AGAINST TOXINS

Listed below are the nine basic Power Recovery Program Detoxification nutrients, along with their appropriate dosages, which are critical in helping you detoxify your body. I've also briefly explained which of your body's detoxification systems each of the nutrients supports. Like the Quick-Start nutrients, these are natural and safe for everyone, and they can be purchased at most supermarkets and health food stores.

Take all of the nutrients listed below in the recommended amounts to help your body improve its ability to get rid of accumulated toxins. Add these nutrients to your Quick-Start nutrients to complete the first two stages of your personal Power Recovery Program. And remember, while detoxification doesn't happen overnight, if you take these nutrients faithfully for several months, you'll almost surely benefit immeasurably in the long run.

Lecithin: 2,000 mg, twice per day. Lecithin is a nutritional "detergent" which is necessary for the proper processing of fats in the liver, gall bladder, and intestines. When levels of this natural detergent are low—this is usually caused by low levels of lecithin-containing foods in the diet or an inability of the liver to synthesize enough bile—fats can become trapped in the liver, inhibiting the liver's ability to remove toxins. Choline, a substance contained in lecithin, is also necessary in the production of the neurotransmitter acetylcholine, and in the construction and repair of cell membranes. *Please note that if you are doing only Quick-Start for Smokers, you do not need to increase the amount of lecithin you are already taking.*

Lactobacillus Acidophilus: 2.5 billion organisms, twice per day. Lactobacillus acidophilus are beneficial intestinal flora which are first introduced into babies' systems through their mothers' breast milk. Since they are living microorganisms, the dosage is given as a recommended number of organisms. The labels on packages of these supplements will tell you how much you need to take to achieve these numbers. Food preservatives, chlorinated water, mercury from dental fillings, and antibiotics taken by prescription or entering the body through meats from animals treated with antibiotics can kill these microorganisms, and reinoculating your intestinal tract with them will strengthen this important barrier to toxins, boost the efficiency of your digestive system, and help protect you from the negative effects of yeast and other harmful flora.

Bifidus: 2.5 billion organisms, twice per day. Bifidus are beneficial intestinal flora which are first introduced into babies' systems through their mothers' breast milk. Since they are living microorganisms, the dosage is given as a recommended number of organisms. The labels on packages of these supplements will tell you how much you need to take to achieve these numbers. Food preservatives, chlorinated water, mercury from dental fillings, and antibiotics taken by prescription or entering the body through meats from animals treated with antibiotics can kill these microorganisms, and reinoculating your intestinal tract with them will strengthen this important barrier to toxins, boost the efficiency of your digestive system, and help protect you from the negative effects of yeast and other harmful flora.

Vitamin E: Up to 400 IU, twice per day. Vitamin E is an antioxidant that works throughout the body to protect your cells from free radicals, which represent toxins in their most dangerous form. Thus, vitamin E helps to minimize free radical damage to tissues and organs.

Vitamin C: Up to 5,000 mg per day, taken in three or four equal doses. Vitamin C is an antioxidant that works throughout the body to protect your cells from free radicals, which represent toxins in their most dangerous form. Thus, vitamin C helps to minimize free radical damage to tissues and organs. *Please note that if you're following the Quick-Start for Smokers protocol, you don't need to increase your vitamin C dosage.*

MSM (Methylsulfonylmethane): Up to 2,000 mg, twice per day. MSM is a sulfur nutrient which supports chelation throughout the body and conjugation in the liver by combining with toxic molecules to render them ready to be processed for excretion.

Alpha Lipoic Acid: Up to 300 mg, twice per day. Alpha lipoic acid is a sulfur nutrient which supports chelation throughout the body and conjugation in the liver by combining with toxic molecules to render them ready to be processed for excretion.

Glutathione: Up to 100 mg, twice per day. Glutathione is a sulfur nutrient which supports chelation throughout the body and conjugation in the liver by combining with toxic molecules to render them ready to be processed for excretion. Glutathione is also one of the nutrient substances required for removal of toxins by the liver.

Glycine: Up to 1,500 mg, twice per day. Glycine is a required nutrient substance for conjugation of toxins, especially fat-soluble hydrocarbons and pesticides, by the liver.

With Quick-Start you've begun to address your neurotransmitter shortages, and with Detoxification you've begun to shore up your body's abilities to process and eliminate toxic substances. These two important steps will be all that many of you need to take. Most of my patients, often even patients with serious substance problems, find that within a few weeks of taking their Quick-Start and Detoxification nutrients regularly they've begun to feel better than they could have imagined. You may very well find that this is the case with you. As your symptoms lessen and you no longer have to struggle against the need for drugs or alcohol, the decision not to return to substance use becomes easier, and your path to recovery clearer.

CONCLUSION

Once you've begun your Power Recovery Program Detoxification nutrients, you're well on your way to eliminating your substance problem. You've taken the important step of putting the "body" back into the recovery of body, mind, and spirit. As I've said elsewhere, nobody has the same substance problem as another person, and nobody's recovery is quite the same as anyone else's. For that reason, it's difficult to give a definite answer to the question of how long you might need to continue the nutrients of the first two stages. But I'd like to reiterate the "rule of thumb" I gave you earlier in this chapter: Most of my patients find that they're comfortable taking both the Quick-Start and Detoxification nutrients together for at least three to six months. If you've stopped the use of all addictive substances, including prescription drugs, alcohol, nicotine, and illegal drugs, you may then legitimately decide it's time to taper off your Quick-Start nutrients taking them only once or twice per day. After a few more months, you may want to reduce the number of doses to three or four times a week, or stop taking them altogether. At this point you may want to taper off your Detoxification nutrients to once per day as well.

If, however, you continue to use drugs and alcohol at any dosage and for any reason, I would recommend that you continue the Quick-Start and Detoxification nutrients until you have stopped using psychotropic substances for several months. The important thing is that you give yourself some time—two or three months, at least—to begin to realize the longer-term benefits of the first two stages of the Power Recovery Program. In the meantime, the next chapter talks about a number of diet and lifestyle changes that you can put into practice to help you maintain your substance-free life.

7

Maintaining Your Newfound Health

In this chapter I'll make several suggestions to help you stay on the path to good health. I'll review the importance of your unique biochemistry and why you need to continue to listen to what your body is telling you during the early stages of your recovery. I'll also add several important tips on how and why you should continue to take your Quick-Start and Detoxification nutritional supplements, and on why paying attention to your diet is very important. While for many of you these suggestions may involve what seem like fairly significant changes in your daily lives, I think you'll find that they all translate to better intellectual and emotional health. Everyone can benefit from the tips that follow.

YOUR BIOCHEMICAL INDIVIDUALITY

Among the primary risk factors for substance abuse which I discussed in Chapter 4 were poor nutrition, exposure to toxins, and stress. One of my patients once asked me, "If these risk factors are present to some extent in almost everyone's life, why doesn't everyone develop a substance problem?" The answer is as simple and as complex as our biochemistry. First, each of us has the same fundamental brain chemistry. Another way to put this is to say that each of our brains functions according to the same biochemical "rules" as everyone else's. And yet each one of us has an absolutely unique biochemical makeup, and that's where the fourth risk factor, genetic vulnerability, comes in. Let me give you an example. Each of our brains produces dopamine. But because we're genetically different from each other, some people require more dopamine than others to feel and behave at their best. Still others have higher needs for serotonin or GABA.

These individual, genetically based variations in biochemical makeup translate to varying nutritional needs. The more dopamine you require, the greater your need for the nutrients your brain has to have to produce it. The same principle applies to each of the other key neurotransmitters which enable us to maintain a healthy emotional, intellectual, and behavioral balance in our lives.

Imbalances can be created by all the risk factors I've listed. That's why it's very important that you make a few lifestyle changes which will help you maintain your biochemical balance and the good health that goes along with it as you work to eliminate the need for psychotropic substances from your life.

I hope it's clear that I'm *not* trying to reduce the differences among human beings to biochemistry. I certainly don't mean to imply that somehow, if all people were able to restore their bodies to a condition of healthy biochemical balance, everyone would feel and think and act the same as everyone else. In fact, I'm saying exactly the opposite. The only way in which we can truly realize our individuality is by restoring the balance which enables each one of us be himself. Psychotropic substances actually prevent us from true self-expression and self-realization by disrupting the brain chemistry that is one of the important elements of our own unique intellectual, emotional, and spiritual character. By eliminating drugs and alcohol from your life, you're taking an important step toward true self-realization. What follows are some suggestions for changes you can make that will further help you maintain your recovery.

MONITORING HOW YOU FEEL AND BEHAVE

One of the things I hope I've accomplished is to make you more aware of the biochemical foundations of your psychological and emotional states. It's very important that you pay close attention to your thoughts, feelings, and behavior, and to what your friends, family, and healthcare providers tell you. These signals are important in helping you know how long you need to continue taking both the Quick-Start and Detoxification nutrients. And so, one of my first recommendations is that, during the next three to six months, as you follow your Quick-Start and Detoxification nutrient regimens, you *keep close tabs on what your body is telling you and actively ask for feedback from those who care about you.*

Let me give you some examples of what I mean. By answering the Quick-Start questionnaires, you identified the neurotransmitter imbalance or imbalances that lie at the root of your substance problem, and you're using the Quick-Start nutrients to reduce or eliminate your need for your substance(s). But what if you've cut down on your Quick-Start nutrients and you feel your mood swings, irritability, sleep problems, or substance cravings returning? What if your spouse or your doctor expresses concerns about your behavior? If you're receiving this kind of feedback from your body and from those around you, it might suggest that you're experiencing a temporary shortage of certain nutrients, in effect reminding you that it might be a good time to increase your Quick-Start nutrients again. If, for example, you've cut back to taking them three or four times per week and your symptoms begin to return, perhaps you should go back to taking them every day, or even twice a day. Make sure your brain has the nutrients it needs to keep your substance cravings from returning.

Here's another example. You might find that you've noticed that taking high doses of a particular nutrient really helps improve your state of mind. Several of my patients have found that they feel and function best when they're taking 8,000 or 9,000 mg of the amino acid tyrosine every day, for instance. Others have found that taking higher doses of B vitamins, particularly vitamins B_3 and B_6, and of vitamin C, helps them maintain a positive outlook and avoid their tendencies to become depressed. Once again, my recommendation is that you listen to what your body and those around you are telling you. If you respond well to a particular nutrient, stay with it. Or, if you want to try an additional nutrient, go ahead.

Here's a story that will explain what I mean. One of my patients was having great success using tyrosine to help her overcome stimulant abuse and restore normal catecholamine production. Her lifelong battle against "the blues" had come to an end. After four weeks of taking both her Quick-Start and Detoxification nutrients, she found that taking 100 mg of 5HTP before dinner and at bedtime helped her relax. Even though her questionnaires didn't indicate she was necessarily serotonin deficient, she had a "hunch," after reading through several of the case histories, that 5HTP might help her, and it did.

Many of my patients find that taking 2,000 mg of tyrosine, along with B-vitamin and mineral supplements, stimulates catecholamine production and helps keep them alert when they need to focus in order to perform well on detailed tasks. Others find that, instead of reaching for the sweets when they feel stressed-out or anxious, taking 50 mg of 5HTP (again, along with B-vitamin and mineral supplements) can restore their serotonin production and improve their mood. And a number of my patients who have turned to or resumed athletic workouts during their recovery swear by the amino acid DL-phenylalanine. They say it not only helps them focus but enables them to work harder with less pain than they would normally be able to do.

You may find that whenever you're facing a stressful period—whether it's an upcoming exam or working overtime or coping with a family crisis—slightly increasing your dosages of Quick-Start nutrients will enable you to avoid turning to drugs or alcohol in order to cope. And if you decide to experiment with other nutritional supplements, especially in the first three to six months of your Quick-Start program, be sure that you add the other supplements to your existing program. Stick to your plan. Do not replace any of your Quick-Start nutrients with others.

The key in all these cases is that my patients are realizing long-term gains by using natural means of enhancing their bodies' own abilities to perform at a high level, and not resorting to potentially damaging psychotropic substances to achieve short-term results. I call this "finding your individual biochemical keys." So don't be afraid to experiment a bit. Sometimes you'll find that if you "tweak" the amounts and combinations of certain nutrients, you'll be able to arrive at optimal *personal* dosages which will enable you to maintain your biochemical balance. Once you've found your biochemical keys, stay with them. They'll only help you improve.

CONTINUING TO TAKE YOUR QUICK-START NUTRITIONAL SUPPLEMENTS

"Why do I have to keep taking nutritional supplements? Can't I get the nutrients I need from the food I eat?" I've heard this question over and over from patients and from audience members at the presentations I give. It's a question I never get tired of answering, because the answer helps to highlight some of the reasons we develop nutrient shortages in the first place.

Let me start with this: Our ancestors used to consume a lot of food. I mean a *lot* of food. Even earlier in our own century, it was not unusual for people, especially working people such as farmers, to consume as many as 5,000 calories per day. They needed this much food to enable them to do the tremendous amounts of physical work they did. One of the benefits of consuming this many calories worth of food is that you also get enormous quantities of nutrients. A 5,000-calorie-a-day diet of the nutrient-rich food our ancestors ate would certainly provide us with the amino acids, vitamins, minerals, and fats we need to support our biochemistry.

But, of course, we don't eat 5,000 calories per day. Except for highly trained athletes in sports such as swimming, long-distance running, and triathlon, most people would gain weight very rapidly if they consumed that many calories. But one of the results is that, while we avoid the gross obesity such a diet would bring about, we also take in significantly smaller quantities of the nutrients that we would get in such a diet. And because our brains still need the same amounts of nutrients as those of our recent ancestors, we've got to find other ways, besides the food we eat, to get those nutrients.

That's where nutritional supplements come in. In an important sense, we need to use nutritional supplements simply to make up for the nutrients our brains and bodies require but which are no longer in our diets. When you reduce the amount of food you eat, you reduce the quantities of nutrients you consume as well, and using nutritional supplements is the most effective way to make up the difference. When you couple this with the fact that the food we eat is itself of less nutritional value than that of our ancestors, the situation becomes even clearer. Nutritional supplements are an important key to maintaining sound biochemical health.

CONTINUING TO TAKE YOUR
DETOXIFICATION SUPPLEMENTS

I can't overemphasize how effective the Power Recovery Program Detoxification nutrients can be in helping you maintain biochemical balance by enabling you to avoid excessive toxic load. Even after you've taken these nutrients for several months or more and the reduction of your symptoms and the feedback from others suggest that you have successfully rebalanced your brain chemistry and detoxified your body, you might consider continuing to take them, even if you lower your dosages. Many of my patients have found that taking a round of Detoxification nutrients once per day, or even three or four times per week, helps them to be sure they're continuing to provide their bodies with the nutrients necessary to stay free of toxins.

IMPLEMENTING SOUND NUTRITIONAL PRACTICES

The heart of the Power Recovery Program is nutrition. I've shown you how to use nutritional supplements as the foundation of your strategy for overcoming your substance problems. But after you've quit using tobacco, drugs, or alcohol, it's very important that you maintain the nutritional head start your recovery plan has given you. Because one fact remains: Poor nutrition is one of the critical risk factors for substance abuse, and if you ignore your diet, you're putting yourself at risk for a relapse, even if you continue to take nutritional supplements.

Let me expand on that last statement. If, for instance, you eat a diet high in carbohydrates and consume lots of "junk food," you may find that you have difficulty maintaining the level of substance-free good health you've been able to achieve by following the Power Recovery Program. By "junk food" I mean food which is highly processed and/or food which contains high levels of preservatives, hormones, and artificial colorings. I know that covers a lot of ground, but the fact is that an overwhelming percentage of commercially available food is just that: junk food. This means that you may have to clean up your diet significantly to hold onto the health gains you've realized. Let me list the foods I consider the chief offenders:

• Vegetables which have been grown with chemical fertilizer and treated with pesticides and herbicides.

• Any meat or poultry products which are produced from animals which have been treated with growth hormones, steroids, and/or antibiotics.

• Many types of deepsea fish, especially tuna and swordfish, which may contain high levels of mercury.

- Almost all commercial breakfast cereals.

- All sweetened drinks, including colas and other sodas, sweetened iced teas, and fruit-based drinks such as lemonade and fruit punch.

- Most canned and bottled fruit juices, including children's "juice boxes."

- Virtually all refined carbohydrates, from bagels to pastas to white bread.

But while one key to avoiding these foods is reading package labels carefully and asking questions of your grocer or butcher, you don't necessarily have to fight what I call the "nutritional war of attrition." By this I mean that you don't have to go through all the foods you currently eat, one by one, and try to figure out whether you should eliminate them from your diet. Instead, take a look at the following recommendations and use them to guide your shopping:

- Buy only organically grown produce.

- Buy only organic dairy products, including milk, half and half, ice cream, butter, and cheeses.

- Buy meat and poultry which make a point of advertising that they are hormone- and antibiotic-free.

- Buy only breakfast cereals which are made from organically grown ingredients.

- Drink lots of filtered or bottled water (as many as twelve to sixteen glasses per day) instead of soda and other heavily sweetened drinks.

- Reduce your carbohydrate intake and eliminate refined carbohydrates from your diet.

- To the extent that you consume carbohydrates at all, eat beans, fresh, non-starchy vegetables, and berries.

The best way to follow these recommendations is to find a supermarket or grocery store which has a produce section devoted to organic fruits and vegetables as well as a "natural foods" section.

CONCLUSION

I've given you a few relatively simple tips to help you maintain the health benefits you've realized and will continue to realize from the first two stages of the Power Recovery Program. Most people find that these two stages are all they need to help them stop their substance abuse and remain substance free. There are some cases, however, in which further treatment is necessary. Usually this happens in people with serious, long-term substance problems, or in people with other serious conditions, such as emotional or psychological problems or chronic physical disorders, which have led or contributed to their substance abuse. It is primarily for these people that I have included Part III: Biochemical Rebalancing. While Part III of this book can potentially be of benefit to everyone who has or has had a substance problem, no matter how severe, you'll find it especially helpful if you're a person who's attempting to deal with the consequences of serious, long-term substance abuse, whether cigarettes, alcohol, stimulants, opiates, or prescription drugs.

Part Three

Long-Term Biochemical Rebalancing

During the Quick-Start and Detoxification stages of the Power Recovery Program, you've focused on your own unique biochemistry. First you identified the specific neurotransmitter or neurotransmitters whose disruption is primary in your substance use. Then you began your Quick-Start nutritional regimen to correct the nutrient shortages that caused or contributed to the disruption. Your next step was to add the Power Recovery Program Detoxification nutrients in order to remove the toxins contributing to your biochemical imbalances and to strengthen your detoxification pathways. These two stages are designed to enable you to maintain natural biochemical balance without drugs or alcohol, and, coupled with the dietary changes I've recommended, they should enable you to stay drug- and alcohol-free.

The reason for the initial focus on your individual biochemistry is this: *You didn't choose your substance of abuse, it chose you.* Now while it may seem a bit farfetched to ascribe the power of choice to a drug, in a very real sense that is what happened to you. Your underlying biochemical and neurotransmitter imbalances were such that there was one primary psychotropic substance or group of substances that satisfied a need or enhanced your mood in just the right way. When you "found" your "drug of choice" (or when it found you), it may have initially seemed like a match made in heaven. In fact, of course, quite the opposite is true.

But while your personal biochemical profile holds the key to the physical causes of your substance use, using a particular substance regularly for a long period of time invariably brings predictable consequences. Unfortunately, these consequences—which range from emotional instability and diminished intellectual capacity to chronic conditions such as cardiovascular disease, gastrointestinal disorders, and osteoporosis, among dozens of others—are all harmful. Fortunately, in almost all cases, they can largely be reversed.

I call these long-term negative consequences of substance abuse cascade effect symptoms. The term *cascade effect* refers to the secondary imbalances that can occur as the body tries to reestablish some sort of biochemical stability in the presence of a disruptive psychotropic substance and an excessive toxic load. Cascade effect conditions often result when depleted nutrient supplies are diverted from relatively low priority bodily processes (such as hair growth) to help shore up high priority processes (such as heart and lung function). It's the body's version of robbing Peter to pay Paul. Except, of course, in the end you really end up paying the piper.

Parts Three and Four of this book, then, are generally organized by *substance* rather than by biochemical deficiency. To complete your personal Power Recovery Program, after you've finished reading this introduction, and after you've read Chapter 8, which contains important background information on biochemical testing, you can choose to go directly to the chapter or chapters dealing with your substance(s) of abuse. In each chapter you'll find: descriptions of many of the specific cascade effect symptoms that are common to your substance; discussions of the biochemical reasons those symptoms have manifested themselves; case histories explaining how individual patients reversed their symptoms through the use of nutritional supplements; and directions for determining which nutritional supplements you should take to correct the secondary biochemical imbalances your substance use may have caused.

By starting your Power Recovery Program Quick-Start and Detoxification nutrients, you've taken the first important steps to a substance-free life. As your need to use cigarettes, drugs, or alcohol is reduced, and as your body improves its ability to detoxify itself, many of you will find that the secondary problems associated with your substance use—from mood swings and anxiety to physical aches and pains to digestive problems— also begin to disappear. The nutritional supplements in the first two stages of my program may provide your body with everything it needs to bring itself back into biochemical balance.

As I've said, however, if your substance use problem is more serious, you may have also developed secondary biochemical imbalances that you need to address, or you may experience occasional relapses, even though you're taking your Quick-Start and Detoxification nutrients. You may find that, while you no longer use nicotine, alcohol, and drugs, you're still experiencing other physical and emotional problems. Part Three of this book will show you how you can achieve the long-term biochemical rebalancing you need to heal the secondary problems your substance use may have caused.

8

Biochemical Testing

A Key to Long-Term Biochemical Rebalancing

It is often difficult or impossible to pinpoint the biochemical consequences of long-term substance abuse without using diagnostic tests,
many of which are available only through a physician. For that reason,
I've chosen to devote a chapter to discussing specific *medical* tests that will
help you identify the biochemical conditions that can cause substance
cravings and that frequently are a consequence of long-term substance
abuse. To put it another way, I'll be talking to you about "a new way to go
to the doctor." I'll be giving you descriptions of the diagnostic tests you
may need to speak to your physician about having performed to precisely identify the biochemical causes of your problems.

TRADITIONAL APPROACHES TO SUBSTANCE PROBLEMS

Many doctors and addictions specialists who take traditional approaches
to substance problems may be unfamiliar with or skeptical about the tests
and treatments that have been so successful for my patients. For that
reason, I'll also explain how you can make sure that you're getting the
medical support you need to enable you to complete your recovery by fin-
ishing the job of rebalancing your body chemistry. Along the way, I'll discuss how so much of contemporary medicine is what I call "shortcut
medicine," meaning that it relies overwhelmingly on the practice of prescribing drugs which are intended to eliminate the symptoms of a condition
or disease, but which usually fail to address the true causes at the cellular
and molecular levels. Shortcut medicine also fails to take advantage of
testing that is available to improve the quality of diagnoses. Psychiatrists

and addictionologists, for example, are notorious for not testing the very organ, the brain, that they're working to heal. A cardiologist who didn't perform extensive tests on the heart of the patient she was treating would certainly be open to a malpractice suit, but psychiatrists and addictionologists routinely bypass available tests and go directly to prescribing drugs for their patients.

It should be clear by now that excessive substance abuse is in fact a condition—usually accompanied by several others—which is largely caused by biochemical imbalances. As you've seen, these biochemical imbalances are, in almost all cases, the result of a combination of the following things:

• Physical, emotional, and psychological stress.

• Dietary insufficiencies.

• Digestive problems, including insufficient production of digestive enzymes, malabsorption, and imbalances among intestinal flora, among others.

• High toxin levels.

• Genetic predisposition.

While most substance abusers will find that the Power Recovery Program Quick-Start and Detoxification nutrients are all they need to overcome their problems, when I treat people with *serious* long-term substance problems, it is often critical that I obtain a "snapshot" of their biochemical health. In other words, I need to know precisely which nutrients are in short supply, what specific toxins need to be removed, what neurotransmitters are out of balance, and what biochemical processes—particularly digestive processes—are not functioning as they should. In order to obtain this information, I use a number of laboratory tests, and the results help me determine the best treatment in each particular case.

This chapter provides information on several of the important tests I use, along with a brief description of each one. In the case histories that follow in subsequent chapters, I'll be referring to the results of these tests quite frequently to explain how I arrive at my diagnoses and treatments. If you choose to work with a physician to continue your recovery, knowing about these tests will help you find a doctor who understands their usefulness.

AMINO ACID ANALYSIS (BLOOD)

Proteins, the foundation molecules on which all life depends, are actually chains of amino acids linked together. They are the most versatile and widely used chemical compounds of life, and amino acids are the building blocks from which they are constructed. Proteins come in an extraordinary variety of shapes and sizes. Some are made up of as few as 15 to 20 amino acids, while others are made up of more than 1,000. They are the main components of almost all tissues of the human body, and most hormones and neurotransmitters are assembled from amino acids. In fact, the primary job of most of the cells of our bodies is the manufacture of proteins from amino acids.

Like every other biochemical process, protein manufacture requires that specific nutrients be available for assembly when they are needed. And since the most important nutrients in the manufacture of proteins are amino acids, shortages of amino acids mean that proteins may not be able to be manufactured in required quantities. As a result, processes which require proteins—including the building and repair of bodily tissue, the transmission of messages by the brain, and the digestion of food, to name just a few of hundreds—can be disrupted, often causing physical and emotional problems.

The Amino Acid Analysis provides information about the levels in the blood of most essential amino acids. Specific amino acid deficiencies are among the most common causes of neurotransmitter imbalances, which in turn cause or contribute to depression, anxiety, mood swings, food and substance cravings, and sleep problems. One of the reasons for the success of the Power Recovery Program is the use of nutritional supplements to bring amino acid levels back to normal and correct the conditions, such as those mentioned above, which were caused or made worse by amino acid shortages.

ELEMENTAL ANALYSIS (HAIR, BLOOD, URINE)

The purpose of an elemental analysis is to determine levels, in the body of the person being tested, of specific chemical elements, or minerals. These tests measure both elements which are essential to life and health (such as zinc and magnesium) and elements which are toxic (such as lead and cadmium).

I use different samples depending on what I'm trying to find out from the test. Blood testing, for example, is best for measuring levels of essential elements such as zinc and selenium, but generally reflects only recent exposure to toxic elements such as mercury or lead. Lead, mercury, cadmium, and other toxic minerals generally disappear quickly from the blood. This means that even though very high levels of these toxins may be present in a patient's body, they become "locked up" in brain and body tissues and do not circulate in the blood. Unless exposure to the toxic element has been very recent, even abnormal levels often don't show up in blood tests, making this type of testing inaccurate for determining whether a patient suffers from long-term heavy metal toxicity.

On the other hand, heavy metals bind readily to hair tissue. In fact, this is one of the ways the body detoxifies itself of heavy metals. Because heavy metals remain locked in hair tissues, testing hair samples gives a much more accurate picture of long-term exposure to these substances than testing either blood or urine samples.

Urine testing can be used to measure levels of both essential and toxic elements, especially where chelating agents, such as certain drugs and the sulfur nutrients in the Power Recovery Program, have been used. Because chelated toxins are often excreted through the urine, this type of testing can detect deep-seated heavy metal residues as they are being removed from the body.

High levels of heavy metals have been linked to many kinds of neurological, psychiatric, and physical disorders. Lead poisoning, for example, has been found to interfere with endorphin receptors, causing laboratory animals to consume alcohol compulsively. Nutrient minerals such as calcium, magnesium, copper, and iron are required for the completion of literally thousands of different biochemical processes in our bodies, and shortages of essential minerals are associated with conditions as diverse as osteoporosis, heart disease, and cancer, to name only a few.

COMPREHENSIVE VITAMIN PROFILE (BLOOD)

While vitamins—and their counterparts, phytonutrients—do not provide energy (as fats do) or serve as building blocks for other substances (as amino acids do), they are indispensable to the success of innumerable biochemical reactions. You'll often hear me say that they function as "cofactors" and "catalysts" in certain processes, which is another way of stating the same idea. Without vitamins and phytonutrients, our bodies' biochemical processes would simply grind to a halt. These substances are required to catalyze the synthesis of all of the key neurotransmitters I've discussed in this book.

Vitamin deficiencies cause or contribute to disorders as varied as scurvy, cancer, and depression, and virtually every patient I treat for a substance problem has at least one serious vitamin deficiency. The Comprehensive Vitamin Profile provides an analysis of blood levels of seventeen vitamins and is indispensable in pinpointing deficiencies of these life-sustaining nutrients.

FATTY ACID ANALYSIS (BLOOD)

Fatty acids (or *lipids*, as fats are also called) consist of a group of chemical substances which perform a variety of extremely important biochemical functions. The membranes of every one of the tens of trillions of cells in our bodies, for instance, are composed primarily of phospholipids, which are one type of fatty substance. Fats are required to create new cells and repair damage to existing cells. The very process of creating connections among neurons in the brain involves the formation of a protective sheath or shield—which is made of another fatty substance called *myelin*—around a portion of the neuron. Low levels of essential fatty acids are associated with impaired brain development, Attention Deficit Disorder (ADD) and Attention Deficit/Hyperactivity Disorder (ADHD), depression, and alcoholism, among many other conditions. A high percentage of the patients I treat for substance problems are deficient in omega 3 essential fatty acids.

The Fatty Acid Analysis measures the levels of essential fatty acids and provides a guide to replenishing them where necessary. Fat is an important component of virtually all brain tissue, and fats are needed to help in repairing damaged tissue. Resupplying the body with required levels of essential fatty acids is a critical component in correcting many of the mood disorders, skin conditions, and gastrointestinal problems associated with the early stages of recovery from substance problems.

ALLERGY PROFILE (BLOOD)

Allergies to food, pollen and dust, and environmental chemicals cause or contribute to a wide range of symptoms, from digestive problems to runny noses to asthma. Allergies are often present in patients who suffer from migraine headaches and Attention Deficit Disorder, among many other conditions. In addition, allergies cause immune system stress by requiring the body to mount defensive responses to the allergens that cause them. These responses are often quite complex, and they frequently take the form of delayed reactions, sometimes taking hours, or even days, to appear. A very high percentage of the patients I treat for substance problems have multiple allergies, and removing specific allergens from their diets and limiting their exposure to environmental allergens are often significant keys to restoring the emotional and biochemical foundations necessary for recovery.

While skin tests can be useful in identifying airborne allergens such as pollen, I've found that an Allergy Profile which uses a blood sample covers a much wider range of potential allergens. Since food allergies, more than 100 of which are tested for in the Allergy Profile, are extremely common among alcohol and drug abusers, this test is very useful in helping people in recovery avoid allergenic foods until their digestive systems are healed and capable of handling them again.

COMPREHENSIVE DIGESTIVE ANALYSIS (STOOL)

I've emphasized what I call the *gut-brain connection* and the importance of a healthy digestive tract, not only in the prevention of and recovery from substance problems, but also in achieving and maintaining good general health. From restoring the proper levels of stomach acid, to regaining the ability to produce the necessary amounts of important digestive enzymes, to re-establishing a healthy balance among intestinal flora, healing your digestive tract can be as important a component of your recovery as rebalancing your brain chemistry. Unfortunately, most physicians are woefully ill-equipped to diagnose and treat these problems, and, in their ignorance, they often downplay the importance of digestive disorders. Doctors often mistakenly inform patients that their digestive problems are caused by emotional disturbances, when exactly the opposite—that digestive problems cause mood swings, cravings, sleep problems, and depression—is far more likely the case. The Comprehensive Digestive Analysis can precisely identify many digestive abnormalities, often before serious symptoms appear.

Digestive disorders are at the heart of so many biochemical imbalances and chronic degenerative conditions that it's virtually impossible to overstate the importance of this test. In many cases, simply correcting digestive disorders enables even patients who have long been troubled with substance problems and other chronic conditions to become symptom-free within a few months.

COMPREHENSIVE ORGANIX (URINE)

Organic acids are metabolic intermediates produced in pathways of central energy production, detoxification, neurotransmitter breakdown, or intestinal microbial activity. Accumulation of specific organic acids in urine often signals a metabolic inhibition or block. This may be due to a nutrient deficiency, an inherited enzyme deficit, toxic build-up, or drug effect.

The Comprehensive Organix Profile provides a view into the body's cellular metabolic processes and the efficiency of metabolic function. Identifying metabolic blocks that can be treated nutritionally allows individual tailoring of interventions that maximize patient responses and lead to improved patient outcomes. From a single urine specimen, the Organix Profile provides important information in the areas of vitamin and mineral shortages, amino acid deficiencies, indicators of vitamin B-complex deficiency, evidence that enables us to assess oxidative damage and antioxidant sufficiency, indicators to assess how effective the body's detoxification processes are, and measures of how well our bodies produce energy and of central nervous system function, among other things.

THE BIOCHEMICAL BASIS
OF THE POWER RECOVERY PROGRAM

The tests that have been described, and several others I'll refer to in individual case histories, are among the many I use in assessing my patients' biochemical health and determining specific treatments and programs of nutritional supplementation. Now let me make an important point about traditional medical approaches, not only to addictions, but to chronic degenerative conditions of all kinds: Many doctors seem to be unwilling to let their patients' bodies do the work of healing. As I've emphasized earlier in this book, if we remove toxins and give the cells of our bodies the nutrients they need to function in a normal and healthy way, they will almost always do so. Given what they need, our bodies will in most cases return us to health without significant medical intervention. Usually, it's not necessary to compound a patient's substance problem by adding more drugs to her toxic load. The Power Recovery Program recognizes that this is true, and I have used and continue to use this principle to achieve unprecedented recovery rates among substance abusers.

Many of the tests I have listed in this section are an important part of my approach to treating substance problems because they help to pin-point several things. First, they show precisely which nutrients are in short supply and need to be added so the patients' cells will be able to resume normal functioning. Second, they help to identify the reasons the nutrient shortages exist, whether they're caused by maldigestion or malabsorption, excessive toxic load, or malnourishment. Third, the tests help identify precisely which neurotransmitters are likely to be in short supply. Fourth, they help identify specific toxins in the body which may interfere with brain function and other biochemical processes necessary in recovery.

Finally, and perhaps most important, the tests emphasize this fact: *Substance problems do not happen in a vacuum.* As you read through the case histories that follow, you'll find, as I myself have found after ordering and reviewing tests for thousands of patients over several decades, that substance abuse doesn't just suddenly appear out of nowhere. Invariably, it's accompanied by other symptoms which are often the result of the same biochemical imbalances which cause or contribute to the substance abuse. It's extremely difficult to overcome a long-term substance problem unless you also deal with the underlying biochemical causes of the problem.

I also want to emphasize one more thing about the case histories which are included in the following chapters and which make extensive reference to the tests I've described: *They are meant only to provide you with a model for seeking further treatment if you suffer from any of the conditions they deal with.* You should not assume that because, for instance, correcting a magnesium deficiency in one patient relieves her of migraine headaches, simply taking additional magnesium will do the same for you. There are often several factors which contribute to symptoms such as migraine headaches, and, in the majority of cases, most or all of them must be addressed before the symptoms subside.

While the Quick-Start and Detoxification stages of the Power Recovery Program are designed to enable most of you to correct key nutritional deficiencies and remove toxins from your body without the need for medical intervention, the Long-Term Biochemical Rebalancing stage does require you to obtain specific information about the nutritional shortages and other conditions that are the causes of your cascade effect symptoms. Normally, this is best done by consulting a physician who recognizes the effectiveness of the type of tests which I introduced in the earlier portion of this chapter.

Most physicians don't use these tests but resort instead to the use of powerful toxic drugs without even, in many cases, knowing the real causes of the conditions they're attempting to treat. But I've found that biochemical testing provides the most accurate and effective basis on which to treat virtually all the chronic psychiatric and medical conditions, including substance problems, suffered by people today. These tests should not represent a court of last resort; quite the contrary, *they are the court of first resort!* They promise to be an important component of your substance-free future.

CONCERNS ABOUT HEALTH INSURANCE

I also want to say a few words about health insurance, because it can have a profound effect on the quality of the treatment you receive. Health insurance regulations vary greatly from state to state, with some states requiring insurance companies to pay for such treatments as chiropractic, massage, and other so-called "alternative" therapies, and others denying payment for such treatments. But even where insurance regulations are relatively flexible and comprehensive, it is often difficult to get health insurance to pay for many of the tests and treatments I prescribe.

Unfortunately, insurance companies often go so far as to dictate to physicians what tests they may order and under what circumstances they may order them when they're trying to diagnose patients' illnesses and disorders. It's not unusual for insurance companies to deny payment for many, if not all, of the tests I recommend.

In my opinion, this is unacceptable. By making financial issues the cornerstone of treatment decisions, insurance companies are playing high stakes poker with patients' lives. There are two reasons for this. First, virtually all of the treatments covered by most insurance companies, especially for substance problems, have been proven to be almost totally ineffective and in many cases detrimental. Second, this type of regulation makes getting effective treatments difficult, in no small part because it means that patients must pay for treatments not covered by their insurance companies out of pocket.

CONCLUSION

The starting point to good health is a strong and balanced biochemical foundation. And the scientific way to understand *exactly* how to achieve this is through testing which reveals the state of your biochemical health. While the Quick-Start questionnaires are helpful in identifying which neurotransmitter imbalances are causing symptoms, and while they have been shown to correlate closely with the results of diagnostic testing, the biochemical tests I recommend are a more precise way of doing this. Even if you choose not to make use of these tests, understanding how they work and what they can accomplish will help clarify the importance of biochemical rebalancing, and if you do not get the results you desire with the Quick-Start and Detoxification protocols, you can come back and do more extensive biochemical testing later on.

9

Overcoming an Addiction to Sugar and Refined Carbohydrates

It's important to note, from the start, that when we use the terms "sugar" and "carbohydrates" we're essentially talking about the same thing. It's also important to note that, when we talk about carbohydrates in this book, we're not talking about foods such as apples or pasta that are composed largely of carbohydrates, but rather about carbohydrate molecules. That's because a carbohydrate of any kind, whether it's "refined" or "complex," is nothing more than a simple sugar or a combination of two or more sugars held together by chemical bonds. This chapter discusses an increasingly pervasive addiction in America: the addiction to carbohydrates. The excessive consumption of carbohydrates, which has come to be known as "carboholism," has grown so dramatically in the past twenty years that it now ranks as one of the most destructive substance abuse problems we're faced with.

UNDERSTANDING HOW CARBOHYDRATES WORK

Carbohydrates (that is, the sugars that make up carbohydrate molecules) are made available for energy very rapidly after they enter our bodies. Carbohydrate digestion begins immediately thanks to digestive enzymes in the mouth, which break down carbohydrate molecules into simple sugars. Most of these dietary sugars and carbohydrates are ultimately broken down or converted into glucose, one of the main sources of energy for almost all of the cells of our bodies. Upon entering the bloodstream, the broken down sugars and glucose can even be reconverted into complex carbohydrates or glycogen and stored in the liver and muscles for short-term (several hours) energy needs through being reconverted back into glucose. Glucose is especially important to our brain cells. The human brain, with its awesome power and extraordinary metabolism, is one of the largest glucose-users in the body. Although it typically makes up only about 2 to 3 percent of our total body weight, our brain typically consumes about 20 percent of the energy our bodies produce from sugars when we are at rest and not exercising our muscles.

Another thing it's important to know about sugar and carbohydrates is that they are highly addictive. This means that virtually all creatures, from humans to birds, love sugar, and when it's readily available, we are compelled by our biochemistry to consume it in large amounts. That's the catch. Tens of thousands of years ago, when our ancestors were hunter-gatherers, before the advent of farming and our ability to store grains (which are an important source of carbohydrates), sugar and carbohydrates weren't available year-round. Our ancestors, during summers, needed to consume as much sugar and carbohydrates as they could and to store it in their bodies as fat so that the calories could be retrieved and used during the winter, when carbohydrates, and other foods as well, were in short supply. The ability to convert sugars and carbohydrates to fat for storage by our bodies was necessary for survival for our early ancestors. This is still the case in many parts of the world where the food supply is inadequate.

Because we have not changed genetically in any significant way for eons, it is still true that body fat is nature's way of enabling us to store calories, and, when we don't have enough sugar and carbohydrates in our diets, or when we have used up the readily available supplies from our last few meals, our metabolism switches to burning body fat, as well as protein, for energy. Typically, our ancestors would gorge on sugar when it was available as fruits and vegetables during summers and monsoon seasons, putting on weight in the form of body fat, on which they could draw for energy during winters and dry seasons. Nature very conveniently provided a way for us to store sugar and carbohydrates as fat so that it would be available to our bodies even if we couldn't find it in the food we gathered. It was absolutely necessary that sugar be addictive so that early humans (and their mammalian cousins) could have this source of energy during lean times.

One of the things this means for most of the world's well-fed modern humans, to whom sugar- and carbohydrate-rich food is in plentiful supply year-round, is that nature's wonderful survival mechanism—the ability to store carbohydrates as fat for long-term calorie requirements, and the ability to build extra lean muscle mass during the active summer months as a second calorie storage mechanism—has caused us to become a nation of overweight people, with all the attendant complications for our health that this causes. Simply put, it is primarily the overconsumption of sugars and carbohydrates that causes obesity. It's not consuming fats that makes us fat, it's consuming an excess of sugar, often in the form of complex carbohydrates, that makes us fat. The current low-fat diet fad represents one of the fallacies in the way most physicians and dietary experts understand how our bodies work, and it's done a great deal of harm to people who are genetically the most vulnerable to sugar and carbohydrate abuse problems.

Our brains need a great deal of glucose to function, and fat can't be converted back into glucose, so in addition to the ability to store carbohydrates as fat and glycogen, we also needed a way to maintain blood glucose levels when dietary sources and storage of carbohydrates as glycogen were used up. In other words, we needed a back-up plan. That back-up plan is a biochemical process called *gluconeogenesis.* This process enables us to actually convert certain amino acids, especially glutamine, into sugar. Now glutamine is present in abundance in much of the animal protein we eat. When we have enough protein in our diets, we also have the glutamine necessary to convert into sugar when we need it. Foods such as pork, poultry, eggs, milk, and cheese—indeed, virtually any high-protein foods—are excellent sources of glutamine.

Most conventional medical doctors, however, misunderstand how carbohydrate, fat, and protein metabolism works. Let me say that it's not really their fault. They—and my experience bears this out—generally received no more than a few hours of education on this subject in medical school, and diet and nutrition were generally scoffed at as having little to do with health. One of the things that the conventional approach to treating virtually all sugar and carbohydrate-related conditions—from Type II Diabetes to hypoglycemia—fails to take into account is that sugar and carbohydrates are, generally speaking, not essential foods. Except for a few of the 300 sugars known as glyconutritionals, carbohydrates represent empty calories designed to be used up immediately or stored for energy as glycogen (starch) and fat.

Let me put this in perspective: The average yearly per capita consumption of refined sugar in the United States today is over 100 pounds, and when that is added to massive complex carbohydrate and junk food consumption, we have the makings of a national crisis. As nutritionally empty calories in the form of sugars and carbohydrates are overconsumed, deficiencies in fats, especially essential fatty acids and phospholipids in lecithin-containing foods, and protein occur. Americans are increasingly overfed with non-essential sugar- and starch-laden foods, while at the same time they are deprived of the essential food, in the form of proteins and fats especially, necessary to stabilize metabolism, heal tissues, remove poisons from their bodies, and synthesize neurotransmitters and hormones, among other things. Over time, this causes people to think, feel, and function badly, and they often resort to using psychotropic chemicals to compensate for the conditions caused by severe dietary imbalances. Another way to express it is that so many of the so-called "sugar" problems afflicting Americans are typically not sugar problems at all, but "protein and fat deficiency" problems. And they're not ever going to be successfully controlled and eliminated unless we deal with the true source of the problem. The following case histories present two of the most common results of overconsumption of carbohydrates: hypoglycemia and Type II Diabetes.

RISA S.: DEALING WITH HYPOGLYCEMIA

Risa S. was a 38-year-old woman who was slim to the point of possibly lacking optimal lean muscle mass. She appeared somewhat nervous. The patient history that she filled out indicated that she had been diagnosed as having an anxiety disorder, and her doctor had prescribed the drug Xanax, a powerful sedative drug that substitutes for the neurotransmitter GABA in our brains. Her patient history also indicated that, in addition to her anxiety disorder, she suffered from mood swings, sugar cravings, fatigue, and difficulty falling asleep.

During our first interview, she mentioned that she tended to snack on "junk foods," especially sugary snacks. When I asked her what happened if she went five or six hours without eating, she replied, "I don't know what would happen. I can't imagine going that long without eating. I don't remember ever doing that. I keep candy bars in my desk at work."

When I questioned her further about this, she remembered times when she was young and went for long periods without eating, and that they had caused her to have headaches. I also asked her if there were any foods that made her feel better. She said, "Well, sugar makes me feel better temporarily, but the cravings always come back. The only thing that makes those cravings go away is protein. When I have a steak dinner, I don't need sugar for hours."

Risa's was a classic case of hypoglycemia, or chronic low blood sugar, caused by protein malnutrition. One of the fairly common cascade effects of hypoglycemia is anxiety. The process by which low blood sugar can lead to anxiety is indirect, and most conventional physicians and dietitians are utterly unaware of it. Low blood sugar is caused by a lack of protein in the diet and not by a lack of sugar or carbohydrates. This fact sheds light on why many conventional physicians provide exactly the opposite treatments necessary to correct hypoglycemia, and mistakenly prescribe powerful psychotropic drugs for their patients' resulting anxiety and other mood disorders.

On the second visit, when I interpreted Risa's test results, her husband was also present. He especially noted that besides having problems with anxiety and ruminating about the future, Risa and he had been attending couples therapy sessions, where she also displayed a tendency to dwell on past resentments and to complain about the fact that he found her to be irritable when he felt there was no justification.

I was certain (and her test results confirmed this) that Risa's symptoms had resulted primarily from the deficiency of a single nutrient, glutamine, and that this deficiency was having a cascade effect. When there's not enough glutamine to perform all of the functions for which this amino acid is needed, then other processes start to fail, resulting in a spate of symptoms. In Risa's case, the shortage of glutamine not only made her incapable of gluconeogenesis, which would have enabled her to keep her blood sugar levels up to normal, but it also translated to the inability of her brain to be able to produce enough GABA, which in turn resulted in her experiencing anxiety. Her doctor, following the typical incorrect conventional medical diagnosis and treatment recommendation, prescribed Xanax, a powerful and toxic anti-anxiety drug. He also failed to diagnose her hypoglycemia, and even if he had, with little training in nutrition he certainly would not have understood how to treat it correctly.

I've talked about the fact that blood sugar is an important source of energy, especially for our brains, and when we don't have enough blood sugar, our bodies must generate it through the conversion of protein into energy, in the form of ATP, by miniature energy factories known as mitochondria within our cells. Risa had already discovered this indirectly, when she had observed that after she'd eaten a high-protein meal, she didn't crave sugar for several hours. When people don't have enough sugar (or glycogen) to supply their brains and other parts of the body with the energy they need, their bodies must have a way to convert amino acids such as glutamine into sugar and/or into ATP for use in producing energy. If this process is overutilized, as you might suspect, there's a high risk that our body's stores of glutamine will be depleted, making this wonderful all-purpose nutrient unavailable for other tasks for which it is needed. The fact that thinner people like Risa don't have an abundance of lean muscle mass (where protein is stored) also usually means that they don't have as much glutamine, which is stored in their muscles as part of their protein reserves, for use in conversion to sugar when glycogen levels get low.

As I've emphasized before, the amino acid glutamine is one of the precursors of the neurotransmitter GABA, a key inhibitory brain chemical that helps us control anxiety. When glutamine is in short supply, as is often the case in thin people, it becomes relatively unavailable for the synthesis of GABA. Thus hypoglycemic people tend also to develop anxiety disorders. They're in effect hit from two sides: They have less than optimal levels of glucose for brain energy and less than optimal levels of glutamine for the synthesis of GABA.

Glutamine is the single most abundant amino acid in the human body, and it is involved in biochemical reactions in virtually every cell in our bodies. It is critical in many important processes, but especially important in the production of energy when sugar is in short supply, in the production of certain inhibitory neurotransmitters, and in digestion. In fact, enterocytes, the cells lining the intestinal tract, actually use only glutamine and not sugar for producing energy. They're the only cells in our bodies that do so. For that reason, glutamine-deficient people also often have gastrointestinal problems, because without adequate glutamine, the cells lining the intestines are deprived of the fuel from which they make their energy, in the form of ATP. Glutamine is often an important component in healing digestive problems.

If Risa had been tested for hypoglycemia, her test results may not have indicated low blood sugar. When glutamine is fed directly into the mitochondria within our cells to produce ATP, it bypasses the conversion into glucose. The result is that blood sugar levels may not be abnormal in test results. So important is this process, that, conversely, if the energy-producing mitochondria in cells are not able to rely on amino acids like glutamine to make ATP, patients can experience hypoglycemic symptoms even when their glucose levels are normal. This baffles most clinicians, who misinterpret normal glucose tolerance test results, and, as with Rita, either ignore their patients' hypoglycemic, anxiety, and gastrointestinal symptoms, or prescribe incorrect treatments. Lab test results are only as useful as their interpreter is knowledgeable, and I often treat referred patients who arrive with lots of valuable abnormal lab test results which were ignored by clinicians who did not understand what these results meant.

There are many ways of producing energy available to the body, and one of the consequences of Risa's high-carbohydrate diet was that the conversion of glutamine into protein was far below her cells' requirements. Since she was thin and, with almost no reserves of fat and protein, she was completely dependent on carbohydrates to keep going. The over-dependency on empty calorie carbohydrates is a condition I call "carboholism." Like all addictions, carboholism is a biochemically driven reliance on a toxic substance in order to function. Carbohydrates, of which most Americans consume hundreds of pounds a year, have long since ceased being beneficial. They are now, literally, poison for most people.

One of the first tests I perform for many of my patients is the blood plasma Amino Acid Test, which identifies amino acid deficiencies. This test is important, because one of the first things I look for in patients with anxiety problems is a deficiency of glutamine. I have often found this deficiency in patients who did not realize that they had an anxiety disorder and that they were actually experiencing the symptoms of hypoglycemia. These people never went for more than a few hours without consuming carbohydrates, and had simply forgotten what it was like to do so.

I also ordered an RBC Minerals test for Risa. I was specifically looking for her levels of the mineral chromium, because chromium is needed by both the serotonin and insulin receptors to function properly. In addition, symptoms of irritability and anger which stem from a disruption of the serotonin process often make anxiety worse, and are sometimes seen as part of the anxiety symptoms. Risa's chromium levels were indeed low, and I prescribed 400 mcg of chromium nicotinate three times per day with meals.

Risa's amino acid assay also indicated that Risa, as I expected, had a deficiency of the amino acid tryptophan. Another test that I had ordered, Metametrix Laboratories' Comprehensive Organix test, revealed that she had low levels of 5-hydroxyl-indole-acetic acid (5HIAA). 5HIAA is a compound that results from the normal process of breaking down serotonin in the brain and body, and the fact that the levels of this metabolite of serotonin breakdown were low confirmed, along with her low tryptophan levels, that her mood instability was not merely a simple GABA deficiency-caused anxiety disorder. I prescribed 300 mg of 5HTP, in the form of a product called Seromel, in order to provide her brain with a key nutrient in the production of serotonin, as well as vitamin-B complex tablets to provide the necessary cofactors to synthesize both of the neurotransmitters in which she was deficient, and 5,000 mg of glutamine powder. All of these nutrients were to be taken twice per day, one hour before breakfast and at bedtime, so they would be well-absorbed. I also prescribed a distilled, purified, concentrated, fish-oil-based Omega 3 supplement, which, among other things, has potent antidepressant effects.

Among the things that most "carboholics" notice is that when they consume sugary snacks they tend to feel better temporarily. They often report that they're more relaxed and less angry after they've snacked on carbohydrates. And it's commonly known now that sugar stimulates the production of serotonin, one of our brain's key relaxing neurotransmitters. The process by which this occurs is fairly complex, and it sheds light on just how intricate our bodies' mechanisms are for making sure we get the nutrients we need for mission-critical processes, especially brain function.

When carbohydrates and sugar are consumed, the pancreas produces *insulin,* a hormone which triggers the transport not only of glucose, but also of fatty acids and many amino acids into the cells of our bodies. The exception to this process is the amino acid tryptophan; during this process, tryptophan remains in the bloodstream and is not transported into the body's cells by the insulin-triggering mechanism. This preserves blood levels of tryptophan so that it remains more available for transport across the blood-brain barrier and thus more available for conversion into serotonin in the brain. This is almost certainly how carbohydrates cause us to relax, or, as some people have put it, to cause us to experience a "sugar haze," a truly psychotropic, drug-like effect. Because her blood levels of tryptophan were chronically low, Risa was inclined to consume large amounts of sugar in an attempt to increase serotonin production, and this contributed to her "carboholism." This frequently leads to clinicians' misdiagnosing carboholism as a form of eating disorder.

The important thing with all of the therapies I prescribe is, of course, results. As Risa took her supplements, she began to notice that she felt less anxious and less angry than she had in years. Her sugar cravings vanished and she was able to go for six or more hours without needing a "carbo fix." Because of this, she was able to gradually taper off her use of Xanax, and within eight weeks she was able to stop using it entirely. She also, at my recommendation, greatly increased her dietary protein and fat intake, and dramatically reduced her sugar and carbohydrate consumption. She gained several pounds of lean muscle mass, and this restored her body's ability to provide glutamine for conversion into GABA and greatly helped to reduce her anxiety. Her nutritional supplement regimen also facilitated her brain's production of GABA and serotonin, and as a result, she and her husband were able to make rapid and significant progress in their couples therapy. She reported that she'd been able to work through and let go of a great deal of what she described as "unresolved anger and anxiety," and both Risa and her husband were able, finally, to enjoy attending yoga classes together. I am happy to be able to say that I have a nearly 100 percent success rate in curing more than a thousand hypoglycemic patients in the more than thirty years I've practiced medicine.

Risa told me that she felt that if she had not made what she called "these biochemical changes," she was sure that she would have continued in the rut she'd been in for years: carboholism, Xanax addiction, and marital strife. She realized that without the fundamental changes in her biochemistry, all the psychotherapy or mediation in the world would have been unlikely to have made the slightest improvement in her life. Like millions of biochemically imbalanced people, Risa was trapped in a vicious circle of addictive foods, medication, dysfunctional behavior, and money wasted on ineffective psychotherapy and/or spiritual counseling. That all changed when Risa took the necessary steps to change her biochemistry.

BENJAMIN B.: OVERCOMING TYPE II DIABETES

Type II Diabetes, like addiction and mental disorders, is not a disease, although all three of these conditions, which are caused by biochemical imbalances, can lead to symptoms and pathology which make them appear to be diseases. Diabetes is an attempt of cells, adapted for eons to spending most of their yearly cycle in a low-insulin/low-carbohydrate metabolic state, to protect themselves from the assault of excess dietary sugar and carbohydrates. Type II Diabetics are simply people who are genetically more vulnerable to this process, because they store fat better than others. In fact, the diabetic genes that provide the body with an enhanced ability to store sugar in the form of fat are often called "famine genes," because our ancestors who had these genes could store large amounts of sugar as fat and were thus better protected against starvation over the long sugarless winters than were those who didn't build body fat as expeditiously.

Typically, Type II Diabetes is treated with blood-sugar-lowering drugs and insulin. There are many pitfalls with these self-defeating treatments. The main problem is that in cases of Type II (or Adult Onset) Diabetes, insulin levels are already too high (the condition is also known as *hyper-insulinism*), and increasing those levels through the injection of more insulin only exacerbates the damage high insulin levels can cause. Insulin is pro-inflammatory, which means that it actually directly injures arteries when produced in excess over extended periods of time. Injectable insulin does this by converting beneficial, artery-protecting Omega 6 oils into so-called "bad fats." While lowering blood sugars does confer some benefit, since it reduces the sugary coating on cells that inhibits their function, lowering blood sugar through injectable insulin or drugs probably does far more harm than good, and there are other ways to lower blood sugar without harming the patient.

Second, treating Type II Diabetes with more insulin, the hormone that is released by the pancreas to enable the transport of sugar from the bloodstream into cells, directly damages cells by forcing them to stuff themselves with more sugar and fat, and this in turn contributes to excessive weight gain, another side effect of the current way we treat Type II Diabetes. The fact is that when we account for all the variables in controlled studies, insulin and drug management of Type II Diabetes probably do not improve longevity or outcomes at all.

Today, since we have an abundance of sugar and carbohydrates year-round, when excess sugar consumption continues beyond healthy levels, the pancreases of most people become unhealthily enlarged when they are compelled to over-produce insulin to force the cells in the body to take in more sugar than they should. Insulin does this by opening up the sugar transport channels (called GLUT4 receptors) on cell membranes. In response, the cells of the body, especially the fat cells, close down the sugar transport channels to protect themselves. This results in the pancreas's further increasing its insulin production to force the cells to open them back up. Eventually, this push-pull game reaches the point at which the cells win the battle, shutting down to the point where there's virtually no amount of insulin the pancreas is capable of generating that can force the cells to accept much more additional sugar and fat. This condition is called *insulin resistance.*

This is the essence of the "battle" that goes on within the bodies of overweight sugar addicts, and it can lead to Type II Diabetes if not checked. The problem is that most doctors and dietitians don't understand that all symptoms and abnormalities reflect the body's attempts to heal and protect itself. This principle of biochemical adaptation is called *homeostasis,* or the attempt to achieve biochemical balance. The biochemical mechanisms of fat storage and insulin resistance are natural adaptations to extremely unnatural conditions, in this case the overwhelming excess of sugar and carbohydrates in our diets that our bodies are unable to deal with. At a time when the body's fat storage mechanism is protectively shutting down because of an excess of insulin, doctors typically prescribe more insulin. This treatment strategy represents a reckless disregard for the well-being of patients, done either willfully or out of ignorance. In either case, it's unacceptable.

One patient who typifies the negative effects of prescribing insulin and drugs for Adult Onset Diabetes was Benjamin B., a 42-year-old male who was 60 pounds overweight and had been diagnosed with Type II

Diabetes. Benjamin's physician had prescribed insulin for Benjamin, and he was also taking other medications that are typically prescribed for diabetics, including the cholesterol-lowering drug Lipitor and the drug Glucophage, prescribed to help lower his blood sugar. Benjamin came to me because a friend of his had been successful in eliminating his Type II Diabetes through the combination of nutritional supplements, exercise, and low-carbohydrate diet that I'd recommended for him. Benjamin was concerned that his doctors had prescribed insulin for him, even though it was clear that it did not work to cure his diabetes but only to "manage" it. The simple answer, which I gave to Benjamin and which I give to all my diabetic patients, is that doctors practicing conventional medicine simply don't understand the biochemical causes of Type II Diabetes, and they're doing what they typically do in situations where they're ignorant of how things work: They prescribe drugs.

The root cause of Type II Diabetes is carboholism, an addiction to carbohydrates. Anthropological evidence suggests that this condition was unknown until the advent of agriculture about 6,000 years ago, an event that enabled us to store carbohydrates for year-round consumption. It is best described as a disease of the microvascular system in which dangerously elevated levels of insulin and blood sugar cause injury to arterioles, among the tiniest of blood vessels in our circulatory systems. When these small blood vessels clog up in response to elevated blood sugar and insulin, the tissues they supply blood to become starved for oxygen and other nutrients, and this leads to the appearance of a host of other symptoms, which in turn leads to the diagnosis of Type II Diabetes. This most often occurs in people who are genetically vulnerable to the effects of high insulin and blood sugar levels.

Benjamin had begun to notice that wounds were not healing as quickly as they had in the past, and he'd begun to experience some numbness in his toes. One of the things that had happened to Benjamin was that he'd gotten a cut on his foot, and he didn't realize he had it because the feeling in his extremities had been compromised. The wound hadn't healed properly, and he developed an infection which was difficult to treat, since his compromised circulation also meant that his body couldn't supply white blood cells and antibodies to the site of the wound to help it heal. Benjamin had read about Type II Diabetes and recognized that he was at risk for blindness because of the shutting down of the small blood vessels that provide blood to the retinas of the eyes, and for eventually having to have fingers or toes amputated because of compromised small blood vessel function in those extremities. These are all things that diabetic persons are at risk for in part because of conventional medicine's mismanagement in the treatment of Type II Diabetes.

After I took a medical history and performed a physical examination, I reviewed the results of some of the basic blood tests that Benjamin had brought with him. I was looking especially for evidence that his kidneys were healthy enough to be able to function normally as he followed my dietary recommendations. I also worked to undo a great deal of the misinformation that he had been given by his family physician about the nature of his condition, especially the idea that it was irreversible. This is an untruth that has permeated medical thinking, and, because it's based on the medical community's not understanding the processes that lead to Type II Diabetes, it's among the most painful and debilitating for patients. The loss of hope is a terrible thing, and the medical community has managed to see to it that its diabetic patients lose hope based on their physicians' ignorance.

Among the important things Benjamin would need to do was, first, begin to follow a diet that was lower in carbohydrates and higher in protein, essential fats, and cholesterol-lowering phospholipids, and, second, begin an exercise program designed to improve his cardiovascular fitness and his ability to burn calories. Benjamin had a number of risk factors for cardiovascular disease, and so I ordered several other tests to make sure that embarking on a physical fitness program would not put him at risk for heart attack. Among those tests was an inexpensive CAT scan of his heart (called a "heart scan"), which revealed that he had no arterial blockages. I also obtained the results of stress tests and EKGs that Benjamin had undergone within the past two years. These tests indicated that Benjamin would be an excellent candidate for a moderately intense exercise program that would keep his heart rate in the 120-beats-per-minute range for at least thirty minutes at a time, three to four times per week.

I explained the basic "game plan" to Benjamin like this: "When we're not taking in as much sugar and carbohydrates in our diets, exercise causes the body to begin to dip into its fat and carbohydrate reserves for energy. This in turn causes the pancreas to say, in effect, 'Hey, I can go back to producing less insulin again, because I see that less sugar is coming into the bloodstream from the diet and that the hungry cells are opening up their sugar transport receptors again to allow sugar to leave the blood-stream.' When we consume fewer carbohydrates and sugars and when we remove them more quickly from the bloodstream due to increased exercise, the pancreas does not need to produce as much insulin as it did before. Once blood sugar levels fall and the pancreas doesn't have to pro-duce as much insulin, insulin resistance goes down. Gradually, this leads back to normal blood glucose and insulin levels."

The fact that Benjamin was taking insulin and Glucophage was an extremely serious complicating factor. (Indeed, treating a Type II Diabetic who has not yet been given insulin or drugs is a relative cakewalk when compared to cases like Benjamin's.) The insulin had been keeping his blood sugar artificially low, so we had to taper his diabetes medications gradually, over time, as his body began to function more normally. With Type II Diabetes patients, it's not high blood sugar levels that are a cause for concern, but rather low blood sugar levels. If Benjamin's exercise and low-carbohydrate diet program were overly aggressive, and his medica-tion and insulin were not tapered at the right pace, he could be at risk for hypoglycemic shock. I explained that he would need to "start low and go slow," and monitor his glucose levels carefully, and that he shouldn't worry if those levels were a bit on the high side temporarily. Because he was a knowledgeable and responsible patient who knew how to manage his blood sugar levels by adjusting his insulin, I had little cause to worry about Benjamin in this regard.

I also explained to him that if it were only a matter of adjusting insulin, exercise levels, carbohydrate intake, and nutritional supplements, everyone's Type II Diabetes could have been cured long ago. I explained to him that the real problem is most often sugar and carbohydrate addic-tion, also known as "carboholism." I had him fill out the neurotransmitter deficiency questionnaires (the same ones that appear earlier in this book), and they revealed that Benjamin had been addicted to sugar since he was young, and that his carboholism was likely in response to his being abused as a child. Carboholism, like many other addictions, can be a way to mask the emotions associated with childhood trauma, and resolving the effects of such trauma is very difficult unless the sugar addiction is first dealt with. As a result of his body's having to produce great amounts of endorphins and enkephalins, he was deficient in three of the five amino acids required to synthesize those neurotransmitters, and I prescribed nutritional supplements to correct these deficiencies.

Benjamin's blood glucose levels slowly dropped over the next three months, and he was able to taper his use of insulin, Lipitor, and Glucophage. Within five months he was able to stop using insulin and medications entirely and, with a few exceptions, he was able to stick with the diet and exercise program I'd prescribed for him. Benjamin was also able to engage in psychotherapy to deal with the results of his childhood abuse as a result of stabilizing his carboholism and bringing his production of endorphins and enkephalins up to normal levels. When I saw him several months later, he was a very different person—20 pounds lighter, calmer, more in control . . . in short, much healthier—than he had been the first time he walked into my office.

A word of caution, though, is in order: Please be advised that if you are a diabetic, especially if you are being treated with insulin and/or drugs, you should *not* try to apply these recommendations here without the assistance of a nutritionally-trained and competent licensed healthcare practitioner. The transition to health and away from drug treatments and insulin can take months, even years, and it can be fraught with serious problems. The successful treatment of Type II Diabetes after you've begun taking insulin is often difficult, and you will very likely need a great deal of support along the way.

CONCLUSION

I've dealt in this chapter with two of the most common effects of carboholism: hypoglycemia leading to anxiety disorders, and Type II Diabetes. Both are directly related to the ways our bodies process sugar and carbohydrates, and both are correctable conditions. They're based on processes I'd like to take some time to review here.

Glutamine makes GABA, and it is the primary amino acid in protein-rich lean muscle mass. Because of this, muscle is the long-term steady source of glutamine to stabilize blood sugar levels. A protein-rich diet is one of the key ways to reduce, and in many cases even eliminate, anxiety problems. It's a key component in getting off of anti-anxiety drugs. Our bodies, and especially our brains, must have sugar in order to function properly, and when there is a deficiency of protein, which is a critical source of long-term sugar supplies, we tend to crave carbohydrates to supply sugar for the short term. When that "emergency" intake of sugar, in the form of high-carbohydrate meals or sugar snacks, wears off—usually within about an hour or so after we eat them—our brains need more sugar, and so we feel the need to consume sugar. This occurs because insulin levels, which have spiked in response to the sugar intake, remain high even after blood sugar levels have gone back down. Thus, protein deficiencies are at the root of sugar cravings, and only the consumption of protein or certain amino acids such as glutamine can restabilize blood sugar levels and eliminate insulin overcorrections due to excessive sugar consumption.

When it comes to carbohydrates, Americans have been misled, especially by our healthcare system. First and foremost, sugar and carbohydrates are highly addictive. Our per capita consumption of more than 100 pounds of refined sugar annually certainly attests to that, and a basic understanding of how our bodies process sugar at the biomolecular level reinforces the validity of the addiction model. Second, carboholism, or sugar addiction, is a direct cause of diabetes, obesity, high blood pressure, depression, and a long list of medical, dental, and psychiatric conditions.

As long as the healthcare system ignores the fundamental biochemical causes of hypoglycemia, Type II Diabetes, eating disorders, and obesity, healthcare consumers will continue to suffer unnecessarily as they're treated with palliative and profitable medications which merely cover up symptoms of carboholism and fail to get to the root of the problem. Add to this the fact that our healthcare system, by in many cases willfully ignoring carboholism, has instead invented other fictitious "causes" of the many conditions carboholism creates, and you've got a perfect storm that results in a significant portion of our population's suffering from an addiction and a spate of resulting disorders that all could be wiped out in a very short time, and without the use of drugs.

As we've discussed, the primary mechanism that our bodies have developed for the long-term storage of calories is fat. The incorrect notion that consuming fat and cholesterol in our diets can cause atherosclerosis has also led to veritable hysteria about high cholesterol levels, and that has resulted in the rise of the cholesterol-lowering drug industry, a shameful scam perpetrated on American medical consumers. Among the utterly false, not to say absurd, conclusions this hysteria has led to is the one that claims that eating fat makes you fat, and eating and being fat leads to heart attacks. A fundamental understanding of biochemistry demonstrates that it is carbohydrates, and not fat, that causes obesity. *Simply put, all of the cardiovascular risk factors I've mentioned here are caused or made worse by carboholism.*

A recent major study in the *Journal of the American Medical Association (JAMA)* compared many types of diets, including high-carbohydrate diets, and found that only the Atkins low-carbohydrate diet lowered diastolic blood pressure as well as triglycerides and other cardiovascular risk factors. So why didn't your doctor tell you? Nowhere else in medicine and psychiatry have I discovered more deception, misrepresentation of facts, and fraudulent advertising and claims than in this area of carboholism and its consequent Type II Diabetes and other spin-off medical, dental, and psychiatric disorders. It's a situation that can only be corrected when people take it upon themselves to become educated to the true state of affairs and to take their treatments into their own hands, with the help of physicians and other healthcare professionals who truly understand how our bodies work and how they can heal themselves if given the right nutritional tools.

10

Overcoming the Consequences of Smoking

Have you ever read the warnings on the package of a so-called "therapeutic" nicotine patch? They caution against continuing to smoke while you use the patches, and they tell you not to use them if you have high blood pressure that is not being treated with medication. You're also warned against using nicotine gum if you're taking insulin for diabetes or prescription medication for depression or asthma. But perhaps the most sinister warnings are those that caution you not to let children have access to either nicotine patches or gum. There's a good reason for this. If by some accident a child who had not built up a tolerance for nicotine should ingest even a small amount of the substance through a nicotine patch, he would almost immediately go into convulsions which would in all likelihood be fatal.

Nicotine is one of the most powerful poisons known. It's so toxic that as few as two or three drops of pure nicotine applied directly to the skin of an average person will kill him within minutes. Toxic doses of nicotine work by causing central nervous system (CNS) depression and paralysis of muscles involved in breathing, leading eventually to death. In lower doses, nicotine can cause high blood pressure, nausea, vomiting and diarrhea, heart palpitations and irregular heartbeat, tremors, convulsions, and CNS overstimulation. There is no known antidote for nicotine poisoning.

How is it that so many people habitually use such a powerful and potentially deadly toxic substance on a daily basis? This chapter deals with the nature of an addiction to nicotine and presents a case history that makes clear how an addiction to nicotine can be overcome.

THE CIGARETTE HABIT

If you're a smoker, or have been at some time in your life, think back to the first time you had a cigarette. If you're like most people, you had to overcome your body's natural revulsion for cigarettes in order, eventually, to realize the effects of nicotine. Almost all of my patients report that they experienced unpleasant side effects, including dizziness, lightheadedness, and/or nausea, the first several times they smoked cigarettes. Their bodies were simply trying to tell them that the substance they were ingesting was toxic, and that they should not use it.

What does this tell us? First, if it weren't for the fact that nicotine changes the way we feel by artificially altering our brain chemistry, most people would not even consider continuing to smoke after experiencing the unpleasant consequences of their first few cigarettes. And many people—those who do not have imbalances which can be temporarily corrected by nicotine—either never try cigarettes in the first place or never smoke again after their first negative experience. That many people do fight through the initial nausea and lightheadedness to continue to smoke will give you an idea of the power of nicotine both to compensate for existing biochemical imbalances and to cause additional imbalances that can be temporarily corrected by further smoking.

Let me recount a story which will help demonstrate how potent nicotine's power to attract is. During the time I was Medical Director of the Tully Hill Hospital, Fred, a 58-year-old chronic alcoholic, was admitted for treatment with a blood alcohol level 2.4 times greater than the legal limit. For the previous two weeks he had consumed more than a fifth of vodka and smoked about two packs of cigarettes per day. During that time, he had hardly eaten a thing.

As part of Fred's treatment, I prescribed round-the-clock supervision, drugs which would prevent seizures and Delirium Tremens during the initial stages of withdrawal, and large doses of many nutritional supplements to help correct the massive acute nutrient deficiencies he no doubt had. By the fourth day of inpatient treatment, Fred was clear-headed enough to carry on a conversation. During our discussion of the treatment plan I proposed to him, I said, "You know Fred, since you're going to stop drinking while you're here anyway, and you've got some pretty serious lung problems, why don't you work on quitting cigarettes, too?" Fred's response was typical. It began with something that translates roughly to "@&%#@!" He went on, saying, "I'm already giving up booze! What are you trying to do? Take away all of life's pleasures?" When he threatened to leave the hospital unless he was allowed full access to his cigarettes, I simply backed off. Instead of arguing with him, I wrote additional orders for specialized nutrients, including amino acids, vitamins, minerals, and essential fatty acids, to restore the neurotransmitters that his nicotine use had depleted.

Within three days, as happens with most patients who follow the Power Recovery Program Quick-Start for Smokers protocol, Fred began to notice that he was losing the urge to smoke, or, as he put it, he was "just burning 'em." When he complained that his cigarettes "tasted like cardboard," another patient who overhead him let the cat out of the bag: "Hey Fred, Doc probably slipped you some of those vitamins for smoking." Like dozens of other patients in the same circumstances, Fred was initially quite upset. He insisted that I stop giving him whatever it was that was making his cigarettes taste like cardboard and causing him to lose the urge to smoke. He was quick to add, however, that he *did* want to continue those that stopped his cravings for booze, and the ones that were helping him get to sleep, the ones that were making him feel good, and especially those that were making him interested in women again.

The story reveals something about attitudes toward smoking. Fred viewed his nicotine use in a very personal way. It was almost as if, by causing him to dislike cigarettes, I had broken some taboo or violated his civil rights. Another of my patients told an anecdote which I think sheds additional light on this point. In explaining his "attachment" to cigarettes, he recalled that, when he was in college, he and his friends used to ridicule the growing evidence of the dangers of smoking.

Those who continue to smoke seem always to be able to find ways to defend their use of cigarettes. Sometimes they take the form of ridicule and gallows humor. Or they might take the form of a complaint that, for instance, those who pass laws against smoking in public are, in fact, violating the civil rights of smokers. Cigarette smokers, like abusers of most substances, often hold an irrational belief that bad things will happen to them if they quit using drugs, while in fact the opposite is true: It's continuing the excessive use of a substance that leads to bad things. Whatever form these defenses take, it's ultimately necessary to get beyond them if you really want to quit smoking, or to maintain long-term recovery from any substance problem. Without your being aware of it, the need to smoke may be shaping everything from your sense of humor to your views on politics.

I've talked about some of the issues surrounding smoking, but the question remains: Just what exactly is a "cigarette habit?" As you might suspect, I define the term by talking about what happens at the cellular and molecular levels when you smoke a cigarette. First, the primary function of cigarettes is to provide a delivery mechanism for the potentially addictive psychotropic substance *nicotine.* Nicotine alters brain chemistry to the point where smokers may develop cravings for the substance, but, unlike most other drugs of abuse, it is not the use of nicotine in and of itself which can lead to the problematic secondary conditions that so often accompany smoking. You don't hear stories about people wrecking their cars and becoming violent because they smoke cigarettes, and smoking has few of the adverse psychosocial consequences which often accompany the use of other drugs. The harmful effects of tobacco are mostly physical and not behavioral. Although even those who use chewing tobacco and other "smokeless" tobacco products can develop localized cancers, particularly of the mouth and throat, as a result of their tobacco use, the most serious harmful effects—from emphysema and lung cancer to cardiovascular disease and heart attacks—which we most commonly associate with tobacco use occur primarily because of the fact that it is smoked.

At last count, more than 100 different toxins had been found in cigarette smoke. And so, while nicotine is the primary addictive substance that keeps smokers coming back for more, the other toxins in cigarette smoke often cause or contribute to the cascade effect symptoms smokers have. In other words, over the long haul, smoking can be a factor in literally hundreds of degenerative conditions.

But the real story of the "cigarette habit" lies in nicotine's effects on brain chemistry. Let me expand a bit on the overview of this topic which I gave in Chapter 5. Nicotine, the primary psychotropic substance in tobacco, is a unique substance, quite unlike any we have discussed so far. Its uniqueness lies in the fact that nicotine disrupts not just one or two, but a wide range of neurotransmitters. By virtue of altering both excitatory and inhibitory neurotransmitters simultaneously, nicotine is able to cause both energizing and relaxing effects on smokers.

While nicotine directly occupies certain acetylcholine receptors, its effects quickly broaden as it disrupts the normal cycles of serotonin, GABA, dopamine, and endorphins and enkephalins. In other words, nicotine involves, to some degree, most of the neurotransmitters which we have discussed as playing a key role in substance problems. After temporarily stimulating acetylcholine receptors, nicotine then rapidly blocks any additional acetylcholine stimulation, either from further use of tobacco or from the brain's own normal acetylcholine production. This makes it, in effect, a self-regulating substance, because continued use actually stops its primary psychotropic effect. I've had patients who smoke tell me that they get a "buzz" in the morning from their first cigarette and then "chase the high" all day. Because nicotine stimulation is not continuous, it provides intermittent psychological reinforcement, which is often a more powerful habit-forming pattern than continual reinforcement.

Because nicotine affects neurotransmitters that are both energizing and relaxing, it does not cause dramatic shifts in mood one way or another and for this reason is not used as a "party" drug. Instead, people generally use tobacco on an everyday basis, or they don't use it at all. There seems to be no middle ground. Although in recent years smoking has gradually lost its once almost universal social acceptance, millions of people continue to smoke regularly without significantly impairing their ability to function in the workplace, at least in the short term.

Most smokers find an optimal standard daily dosage with which they are comfortable and continue to smoke at that level. Smokers who quit and then resume smoking usually return to their personal dosage very quickly. In fact, reducing the number of cigarettes smoked per day or temporarily stopping smoking is, as those of you who smoke know, very difficult. When you're asleep, nicotine levels in your brain drop off, and the acetylcholine cycle, along with those of the other neurotransmitters affected by nicotine use, all phase into the withdrawal state. By morning, they are ready once again for nicotine.

If you quit smoking "cold turkey," nicotine levels in your brain fall dramatically. As with other drugs, this causes your brain, which had learned to function in the presence of nicotine, to have to regain the ability to function without it. The result can be unpleasant, though generally harmless, withdrawal symptoms, including irritability, impatience, hostility, anxiety, depressed mood, difficulty concentrating, heart palpitations, gastric disorders, restlessness, decreased heart rate, increased appetite, and weight gain. This wide array of physical, psychological, and behavioral withdrawal symptoms is the result of nicotine's effects on so many neurotransmitter systems.

CASCADE EFFECT CONDITIONS RESULTING FROM LONG-TERM SMOKING

Many of smoking's long-term cascade effect symptoms—including high blood pressure, lung disorders, and cardiovascular disease—are well known. But there are some of which you might not be aware. Both the commonly understood and lesser known conditions are discussed below.

High blood pressure is one of the most well known of smoking's cascade effect conditions. Nicotine is a *vasoconstrictor.* This means that it causes the tiny muscles around blood vessels to squeeze harder on the blood vessel itself, thus causing a rise in blood pressure.

Breathing difficulties, including *shortness of breath,* represent another cascade symptom that people commonly associate with smoking. Toxins in cigarette smoke irritate and in many cases destroy the cells and connective tissue of the tiny air pockets that line the interior of the lungs. The resulting loss of surface area decreases the lungs' ability to exchange oxygen for carbon dioxide, which in turn can cause breathing difficulties.

Nicotine affects catecholamine receptors in the muscles of the heart, causing the heart to become overstimulated and irritated. If the irritation is severe enough, *heart arrhythmia* or *palpitations* can result. This condition can result in an increase in the risk of heart attacks in people who smoke.

The name *leukoplakia* refers to tiny pre-cancerous lesions in the mouth. The lesions are often difficult to see unless a thorough examination of the mouth is done. If left untreated, these lesions can lead to cancer, particularly of the throat and larynx.

Raynaud's Syndrome, also worsened by the fact that nicotine is a vasoconstrictor, is characterized by numbness and coldness in the fingers and toes. It is a cascade symptom of smoking that results from decreased blood circulation to the extremities.

Smokers can also suffer from *high carboxyhemoglobin levels.* The carboxyhemoglobin level in the blood indicates the degree of carbon monoxide poisoning in the blood, or, more specifically, the amount of hemoglobin that is tied up by carbon monoxide and thus prevented from carrying oxygen to bodily tissues. High carboxyhemoglobin levels mean that the supply of oxygen in the blood is lower than it should be.

High cadmium levels can also be a problem for smokers. Cadmium, a heavy metal, is used in the manufacture of many brands of cigarettes. It can accumulate in the bodies of smokers over time. Heavy metals do most of their damage at the cellular level by chemically bonding to the sulfur molecules of several amino acids, rendering the proteins in which they occur useless. Since amino acids are the building blocks of proteins, and proteins are the most versatile and widely used chemical compounds of life, heavy metal toxicity can often seriously compromise biochemical function.

These conditions are discussed in more detail in the following case history. I want to emphasize that this case history is meant to provide you with a *model* for seeking treatment and correcting any cascade effect symptoms your smoking or nicotine use may have caused. These secondary conditions, many of which can become very serious if left uncorrected, develop as a result of many factors, including genetics, stress levels, diet, and exposure to toxins. The best way to determine the precise biochemical causes of cascade effect symptoms is to speak with your physician about having biochemical testing done by a qualified lab.

JOAN R.: LOOKING FOR HELP IN ALL THE WRONG PLACES

Joan R. was a 34-year-old woman who came to me for help in stopping smoking. For the past twenty years, she had smoked, in her words, "more than a pack a day, but I guess I don't want to know how much more, because I never really added them up. But it's less than two packs, that much I know."

She'd been trying to quit since, in her words, "about two minutes after I started. I'd walk around saying, 'God, what a stupid idiot you are to take up this filthy habit,' but beating myself up like that didn't seem to do much good either, so I stopped it. It seems like, regardless of what I do, I just can't quit. Can't even smoke less, for that matter." And it's not as if, like millions of other smokers, Joan hadn't tried. Her list of stop-smoking strategies included hypnosis, acupuncture, nicotine gum and patches, antidepressant drugs, and Clonidine. She had also participated in two separate programs sponsored by the American Heart Association, and she'd gone "cold turkey" twice, only to resume smoking within weeks.

Her main concerns, which had come to focus on health and quality-of-life issues, had emerged in the past several years, particularly since she watched as her father, who was also a smoker, died of lung cancer. "I know he'd want me to stop," Joan said with tears in her eyes. After she had regained her composure, she admitted that her appearance was also an important concern. "This may sound trivial, but people have always guessed that I'm younger than my actual age. Now, I don't know. My face is getting wrinkles that shouldn't be there. I'm starting to look my age. I know my husband and our friends notice it. They say cigarettes can do that."

I was not Joan's primary care physician. A friend who I had helped overcome an alcohol problem had recommended me to Joan, and Joan was determined to give it "one last try." She explained that several of the methods she had tried in the past were suggested by her primary care physician, but that she really didn't think the doctor was paying attention to what Joan was trying to communicate about her problem. "My doctor—and don't get me wrong, she's very good in other ways—well, she just didn't seem to understand how serious my smoking problem was to me. She kept saying things like, 'Well, we've got a lot of options here, so let's try the patch one more time, and if that doesn't do it, we can go on to something else.' It was like she was going through some checklist and not really looking at *me*, at what *my* particular problem was."

When she mentioned the word "checklist," Joan was probably closer in her assessment of her doctor's method of determining treatment than she realized. Her primary care physician was a member of an HMO. There is, indeed, a list of approved treatments for stopping smoking, and Joan's physician may well have been running down the list of those treatments. Unfortunately, as Joan and millions of other smokers have discovered, every one of the approaches on most HMOs' lists of approved stop-smoking treatments which has been clinically studied has proven to have disappointing outcomes.

Joan was being treated for several conditions which almost certainly either resulted directly from her smoking or were made more serious because she smoked. She had high blood pressure and was taking medication to bring it down. She also complained of shortness of breath, and she said that she sometimes had difficulty breathing. Her doctor had diagnosed her breathing difficulties as asthma and had prescribed two different kinds of inhalers to treat the symptoms. Joan needed to use them several times per day, though, she said, "There are times when it seems like I'm puffing away on those inhalers as often as I'm puffing cigarettes."

Joan also said that she sometimes felt heart palpitations—which are serious symptoms and not to be dismissed lightly—though she had not told her physician about them because, as she put it, "I've been having them for years. I guess I got so used to them that I don't even consider them abnormal." She also occasionally experienced some numbness and coldness in her fingers and toes. When I questioned her further about this, she admitted that it got "pretty bad" sometimes. It turned out that "pretty bad" meant that she was extremely sensitive to cold, and that if, for example, she picked up a cold object such as an ice cube tray, her fingers would quickly turn blue. This condition, not uncommon in smokers, is known as Raynaud's Syndrome. I questioned her about her exercise endurance and other cardiovascular and lung-related symptoms. She admitted that she was no longer able to exercise the way she had been able to even four or five years ago.

After I had interviewed her, I performed a routine physical examination. Her breath sounds, harsh and characterized by wheezing, were typical of a smoker. I also discovered several tiny white lesions, known as *leukoplakia,* near the back of her mouth. She was surprised that I took the trouble to look into her mouth: "I thought doctors only did that if you had a cold or sore throat or something like that." The remainder of her physical exam revealed no other abnormalities.

After I had completed Joan's physical, I discussed my approach to substance treatment and recommended that she start immediately with the Power Recovery Program Quick-Start for Smokers and Detoxification nutrients. In addition, I prescribed vitamin C, in the form of a powder, which Joan would dissolve in fruit juice and "swish" around her mouth before she swallowed. Antioxidants such as vitamin C have been shown to be effective in reversing leukoplakia, which is a pre-cancerous condition, in smokers. I also recommended that she take 1,000 mg of the amino acid taurine, in the form of magnesium taurate, three times per day, to treat her intermittent heart palpitations. Both magnesium and taurine are usually effective in reducing heart palpitations. Potassium also helps to reduce heart palpitations, and all three supplements are helpful in reducing high blood pressure, so I encouraged Joan to purchase a potassium-based product called Nu-Salt(r) at the grocery store and use it on her food.

I don't resort to scare tactics, such as ranting about the increased risk of cancer and heart disease, when I'm treating patients who are trying to stop smoking. In practical terms, this approach almost never works, and I was happy to hear that Joan's doctor had not used it. Most smokers are fully aware of the risks they run. But even more important, scare tactics, especially when they are used by a doctor, tend to upset patients, and the resulting stress further depletes their already reduced supplies of key neurotransmitters. This, in turn, often leads them to increase their substance use to compensate for the deficiency. Unfortunately, this scenario—with doctors literally scaring their patients into greater substance use—is repeated thousands of times daily, because many physicians and clinicians have no idea of the effects of stress on brain chemistry. They are in fact acting out a persecutorial role, filling the role of "enabler" in a codependency relationship. Conversely, my conveying hope to patients through educating them and sharing the excellent clinical outcomes my patients achieve tends to accomplish just the opposite: It lessens stress and helps reduce the depletion of neurotransmitters.

I then recommended that Joan at least get a chest X-ray, pulmonary function tests, and an EKG to more carefully explore the possibilities of lung or heart disease. I also recommended blood testing, including routine chemistries and CBC (Complete Blood Count), an Amino Acid Analysis, a carboxyhemoglobin level test to measure her carbon monoxide levels, a test to measure intracellular RBC (within red blood cells) selenium, magnesium, and zinc levels, and a blood cadmium level test. (The toxic element cadmium is a contaminant in commercial cigarettes.) I forwarded these recommendations in a letter to Joan's primary care physician.

All of the tests I'd requested, except the chest X-ray and EKG, were promptly determined to be inappropriate, unusual, and uncustomary, and coverage was rejected by the HMO of which Joan's doctor was a member. Joan's physician, because she is an employee of the HMO and not free to make her own choices about treatments such as this, could do nothing about the HMO's decision. In an important sense, Joan's regular doctor does not work for her patients but for a corporation, which sets limits on many things, from how much time she can spend with her patients to what tests she can and cannot order. By making financial issues the cornerstone of treatment decisions, HMOs are, as I've said, playing high stakes poker with patients' lives. Joan was forced to pay out of pocket for the tests which were not covered by her insurance company. On the bright side, she would be saving more than $200 per month by quitting smoking, and at that rate she'd have paid for all of her treatments in less than six months.

Joan's next appointment with me, three weeks later, was for the purpose of reviewing the blood tests I had ordered. In the meantime, she had been taking the Quick-Start for Smokers and Detoxification nutrients along with magnesium taurate and potassium. We first reviewed her Elemental Analysis test, which provides, among other analyses, information on a person's cadmium level. Joan's cadmium level was 3.5 parts per million, which was listed on the lab report as toxic for a nonsmoker, but at the high end of the normal range for smokers. A significant proportion of cigarettes' long-term toxicity takes the form of cadmium poisoning, because cadmium can remain in the body for years after smoking ceases. I recommended that she double the amount of sulfur nutrients she was taking as part of her Power Recovery Program Detoxification, because they were the key to removing the cadmium from her body through chelation. I also suggested that Joan be retested for cadmium toxicity in about six months so we could monitor how well her body was able to remove this substance.

Joan's carboxyhemoglobin level was also in the toxic range for nonsmokers, but at the high end of the normal range for smokers. Joan's chest X-ray, although normal, did show evidence of overexpansion of the lungs. Because of a loss of lung surface area across which inhaled oxygen passes into the bloodstream, and because of lowered blood oxygen levels, smokers often must compensate by breathing more deeply than nonsmokers. I explained that this was one of the early warning signs of emphysema, but that if she could restore her lungs to more nearly normal functioning, she was not in danger of developing the condition.

Joan's Amino Acid Profile showed moderate deficiencies of both tryptophan and tyrosine, and a severe taurine deficiency. Taurine is necessary to maintain normal electropotential in the cells of the muscles of the heart, brain, and nervous system, and it was not surprising, given the low taurine levels this test revealed, that Joan suffered from heart palpitations. Taurine helps to regulate the calcium and magnesium levels both in and outside of cells, and those in turn help in the avoidance of heart palpitations. While Joan's EKG was essentially normal, it did show several benign Premature Ventricular Contractions (PVCs) per minute. This abnormality was not serious enough to warrant treatment. Her Quick-Start for Smokers nutrients included both 5HTP (which is made from tryptophan during the manufacture of serotonin) and tyrosine, and she was taking magnesium taurate as well, so her levels of these nutrients could be expected to return to normal over several weeks or months.

Joan's RBC selenium and magnesium levels were moderately low, and her magnesium and taurine deficiencies were likely contributors to the PVCs found on her EKG. Selenium is important in helping to maintain the potency of vitamin E, which in turn helps promote the antioxidant activity of other nutrients, such as vitamin C. This is very important as a cancer prevention measure in smokers and, in Joan's case, in helping vitamin C reverse her leukoplakia. I always recommend that smokers take high doses of antioxidants, including vitamin C and vitamin E, as well as the Detoxification nutrients, even after they have stopped smoking.

Joan's recovery was gradual. She was worried and reluctant to quit smoking entirely because, as she put it, "The last time I quit, I got real moody, and I gained weight, and I don't want that to happen again." She was quick to add, however, that she was taking her nutrients "faithfully." At her six-week appointment, she was down to seven cigarettes per day, and her demeanor had changed noticeably. She was more confident and seemed less self-critical. Joan smiled when I mentioned that she didn't seem to have gained any weight. Finally she said, "I'm ready to quit, I think, but I'm not sure quite how to go about it."

We discussed her options and arrived at a strategy that Joan was comfortable with. She decided to give acupuncture another try, and she set the date of her first acupuncture appointment as her stop-smoking date. Although she had tried acupuncture before, I pointed out to her that, while acupuncture can be a very effective stop-smoking method, if the patient's biochemistry remains seriously out of balance, the treatment has very greatly reduced chances of long-term success. In Joan's case, I felt that she had restored her biochemical health to the point where she was "ready to succeed," and that her chosen strategy was a good one.

When she returned for a follow-up visit a month later, Joan was smoke-free. "Well, I'm a born-again breather," she said with a smile. "I'm still not sure I believe it, but I honestly didn't have any withdrawal symptoms at all. To tell you the truth, by the time I got to the acupuncturist I knew this was it. I knew I was going to quit." She got a serious look on her face, then she said, "Tell me something. Did I really need the acupuncture at all?" I kept quiet, but I couldn't suppress a little smile. Far be it from me to question my patients' successes.

Joan found that after three months she could taper her Quick-Start nutrients to the point where she was taking them only once per day, instead of three times daily. Six months later, when she returned for another follow-up visit, retesting showed that her levels of magnesium, selenium, tryptophan, tyrosine, and taurine were all back within normal limits. Her Elemental Analysis test revealed that her cadmium level was so low that it was undetectable. Her EKG was normal, and she reported that she had noticed a marked increase in the amount of exercise she was capable of performing without becoming winded. There was no evidence of leukoplakia, and her breathing had cleared up significantly. The glow that emanated from her reflected both the pride she felt in being able to quit smoking and the new vitality that resulted from her improved physical condition.

CONCLUSION

In the past there have been debates about whether nicotine is truly an addictive substance. Those who claimed that it wasn't pointed to the fact that many people who smoked did not become addicted. Of course, there can no longer be any debate about the fact that nicotine is a potentially addictive substance. What was not well understood until fairly recently is the fact that the habitual use of a substance like nicotine really depends on the biochemistry of those using it. All substance problems are "two-way streets," so to speak. That is, many people can use psychotropic substances occasionally, without becoming addicted to them, because their biochemistry does not make them susceptible. Others who have biochemical imbalances for which substances temporarily compensate may develop a need to use substances, and continued use can actually make the imbalances worse. This reinforces the need to use the substance.

But if the addictive nature of nicotine has not been well understood until recently, there has been—for the past thirty-five years at least—no question about the health hazards posed by smoking. Even the tobacco companies have plastered warnings all over cigarette packs. I've dealt with several of the more common conditions that can result from smoking in this chapter, but the important thing is that I've given you a model for pursuing treatment if you're a long-term smoker.

The Power Recovery Program gives you the tools you need to quit smoking by correcting the biochemical imbalances that keep you coming back to cigarettes. Because it restores biomolecular health, it actually enables quit-smoking strategies such as acupuncture to work. And it can help you correct the cascade effect symptoms that have resulted from your tobacco use. But perhaps equally as important, the Power Recovery Program gives you the tools you need to avoid becoming one of the "victims" of "big tobacco."

Joan R.'s case history is meant to provide a model for smokers who are looking for proven, effective ways to reverse the conditions associated with smoking. But I want to emphasize that, if you're a long-term smoker who has found some success with the Quick-Start and Detoxification stages of the Power Recovery Program, but would like to take your recovery further, you will benefit greatly from finding a physician who can work with you to order the diagnostic tests that will enable you to complete your successful recovery. For people recovering from the cascade effect conditions of serious long-term substance problems, testing is the proven path to correcting biochemical imbalances.

11

Overcoming the Consequences of Alcohol Abuse

One of the things I try to recognize when treating patients for any substance problem is that every case is unique and that each patient's problem is, in the end, a personal one. The important thing is not how much productivity in the workplace is lost because of substance problems, or how much money is spent annually in treating substance problems. While virtually all of my patients are aware of some of the statistics surrounding substance use, in the final analysis, their concerns are personal. All of my patients who abuse alcohol are interested in reversing the effects of their alcohol use and restoring their health, reducing or eliminating the amount of alcohol they consume, and preventing relapse.

Just as each individual is biochemically unique, each substance problem differs from every other one. Discussing the topic as if there are across-the-board "cures" for alcoholism or cocaine abuse or a cigarette habit is not only to falsify the problem but to do a great disservice to those who struggle with substance problems and to their families. Yes, it is, in a sense, "society's problem." But the solution can only be found by the individuals who make up that society.

The point of what I've just said will become clearer in the following case histories. Although both Sam and Sarah abused alcohol, their biochemical "reasons" for doing so were very different. Any attempt to treat them both with the same protocols would be doomed to failure, as every "one-size-fits-all" approach to substance abuse treatment is.

CASCADE EFFECT CONDITIONS
RESULTING FROM LONG-TERM ALCOHOL ABUSE

There are quite a few cascade effect conditions that the body can experience in response to prolonged alcohol abuse. These conditions are briefly discussed below.

Hyperinsulinemia (which means "excessive production of insulin") is a condition in which the body overproduces insulin, usually in response to excessive consumption of carbohydrates. Hyperinsulinemia is an early warning sign of Adult Onset Diabetes and is reversible by decreasing the consumption of sugars and carbohydrates. The consumption of alcohol worsens hyperinsulinemia. Treating hyperinsulinemia with insulin injections, as many doctors do, actually speeds up the vascular complications, including heart disease and stroke, which are associated with diabetes.

Liver disease is a well known cascade effect condition of long-term alcohol abuse. The liver must bear the brunt of detoxifying our bodies of alcohol. As a result, a person who chronically abuses alcohol is at risk for *cirrhosis* (scarring of the liver) and developing *fatty liver* (where functioning liver cells are replaced by fat cells).

Long-term alcohol abuse also *heightens the risk of osteoporosis.* Alcohol has a diuretic effect; that is, it causes the body to get rid of fluids. One result of this is that it tends to deplete minerals, including calcium, as it draws fluids from the body. This can cause demineralization of bones, leading eventually to osteoporosis.

Alcohol disrupts the normal production of several neurotransmitters, including serotonin (which is converted to melatonin) and GABA. Both of these neurotransmitters work to induce and maintain normal sleep. So alcohol abuse can result in *sleep disorders.*

The consumption of alcohol can cause blood vessels in the brain to dilate, causing *migraine headaches.* Also, already occurring migraine headaches can be made worse by alcohol use.

High blood pressure can result from alcohol abuse. Alcohol depletes the body of essential nutrients that aid in maintaining normal relaxation of the tiny muscles around blood vessels. In the absence of these nutrients, the muscles tend to squeeze harder, raising blood pressure.

In addition to its disruptions of neurotransmitters important to normal sleep, alcohol also causes imbalances in neurotransmitters which help us to maintain a healthy emotional state. In many cases, this leads to *anxiety* and *depression*.

And alcohol disrupts the normal production of endorphins and enkephalins, the brain's natural painkilling neurotransmitters. This actually causes the brain to lessen its production of these neurotransmitters. Long-term alcohol abuse can cause the depletion of these substances, leading to *extremely low tolerance for pain.*

Among the most prevalent cascade effect symptoms of long-term alcohol abuse are *gastrointestinal disorders,* often lumped by physicians under the catchall names of *Irritable Bowel Syndrome* and *Acid Reflux Disease.* In fact, conventional medicine has invented numerous diagnostic labels but has paid almost no attention to their underlying causes, among the most frequent of which is alcohol abuse. Better diagnostic terms, terms which actually reflect the underlying causes of the symptoms, include the following: Leaky Gut Syndrome, maldigestion (the underproduction of digestive enzymes), Intestinal Bacterial Infections, and Intestinal Yeast Overgrowth. When alcoholic people complain of gastrointestinal symptoms to their physicians, they are almost always treated only for the symptoms, while the true causes of their symptoms remain unchecked. Let me briefly talk about some of these conditions.

The term *Leaky Gut Syndrome* refers to a condition in which undigested molecules of certain foods slip through the walls of the intestine into the bloodstream, where they appear to our bodies' defenses as foreign substances and cause an immune system response. Leaky Gut Syndrome can be worsened by maldigestion, or the underproduction of digestive enzymes. In such cases, food molecules are not broken down into small enough parts to be absorbed normally through the cells of the intestinal walls, and they appear to the immune system to be foreign substances that need to be attacked. The underproduction of digestive enzymes can also cause undigested food to remain in the intestine, where it is fermented by gas-producing microorganisms, causing bloating, gas, and intestinal pain. In addition to these potential causes of Irritable Bowel Syndrome, many alcoholic people have bacterial infections which can cause such symptoms as heartburn and upset stomach. I discuss these symptoms in detail in the case histories that follow.

Finally, most people who have abused alcohol for many years also have serious *nutritional deficiencies,* particularly of the amino acid glutamine, the mineral magnesium, and the Omega 3 fatty acids. I deal with several of these in the case histories that follow.

The above-described conditions are discussed in more detail in the following case histories. I want to emphasize that these case histories are meant to provide you with a *model* for seeking treatment and correcting any cascade effect symptoms your alcohol abuse may have caused. These secondary conditions, many of which can become very serious if left uncorrected, develop as a result of many factors, including genetics, stress levels, diet, and exposure to toxins. The best way to determine the precise biochemical causes of cascade effect symptoms is to have biochemical and other diagnostic testing done by a qualified lab. These tests can be ordered by any qualified primary physician.

SAM F.: DOING MORE THAN JUST HANGING ON

Sam first walked into my office nearly three years ago. At the time he was 51 years old. His wife, Doris, accompanied him on his first visit for a one-hour consultation. Doris had heard of my work and had recommended that Sam come to see me. I involved Doris extensively in Sam's treatment.

Sam was a marketing executive at a mid-sized company, where he'd worked for sixteen years. He spoke of his children with a father's pride. His 16-year-old daughter had been accepted to an excellent college under an early admission program. His son, aged 13, excelled in sports. As an eighth grader, he'd played on the high school's junior varsity basketball team. Sam and Doris had been married for nineteen years.

Sam's treatment for alcoholism had included three inpatient rehabilitations, averaging three weeks each, and numerous outpatient therapies, which typically lasted for about three months and emphasized counseling, with Sam attending group therapy meetings at least twice a week. Sam also attended AA meetings. Doris emphasized that despite these efforts, Sam continued to relapse.

Sam had no apparent denial of his alcoholism. He was functioning fairly well, but he was clearly worried that his drinking was getting out of control again. His current pattern was to consume seven or eight drinks a day for a period of three or four days and then to stop drinking. His periods of abstinence ranged from two or three days to a week. He did not experience serious withdrawal symptoms during the times he was not drinking, probably, he thought, because he had not yet returned to drinking extremely heavily. He recognized that he was "playing with fire," as he put it. In other words, he was in an early phase of another relapse cycle, and he didn't hesitate to admit it.

Sam was also aware of the consequences of his alcohol problem: "Well, my company has pretty much wasted, I'd say, easily $75,000.00 on my treatments, and not one of them has had any lasting effect. And I don't want to think about how many times I've been passed over for a promotion." He added that he'd had two DWI convictions and had difficulty getting auto insurance. Sam looked away from Doris when he talked about the suffering he'd caused his family. He summed his drinking up this way: "You know, it feels like every day I'm just struggling to hang on. I keep wondering when I'm going to lose my grip. I want to do more with my life than just keep hanging on."

It was interesting, I pointed out, that Sam didn't list any physical problems associated with his alcoholism. Patients whose treatment, like Sam's, had been heavily weighted toward the psychosocial and spiritual aspects of alcoholism often did not fully realize that they had serious physical problems as well. In fact, Sam did have several physical problems which he had not mentioned because, as he put it, "What do they have to do with my drinking?" Sam was about 30 pounds overweight, and when I asked him about his eating habits, a recurring theme in his answer was *carbohydrates.* He and Doris openly discussed Sam's lack of sex drive. Sam was also taking medication for high blood pressure, and he was a pack-a-day smoker.

As Sam provided more details about his treatment history, it became clear that he had suffered physically, and not just because of the alcohol he consumed. As a result of the well-intentioned but nonetheless inappropriate prescribing practices of several doctors, Sam had been taking four psychotropic prescription medications: Campral, Ritalin, Prozac, and Xanax. In addition, he was taking medication for high blood pressure, and he had a "puffer" or "inhaler" for the chronic bronchitis that had resulted from his cigarette smoking, which he described as "actually heavier than a pack a day" when he was drinking. Sam was also taking Tylenol for his arthritis symptoms and Lomotil for the diarrhea he experienced frequently. Sam had had two gastroscopies, stomach examinations in which a fiber optic tube was inserted into his mouth and down into his stomach. Both were normal. He had also undergone three expensive colonoscopies for irritable bowel symptoms and blood in his stool. These too showed no problems.

Sam's scores on the Quick-Start questionnaires had indicated that he was very probably serotonin-deficient and probably GABA-deficient as well. After explaining the Power Recovery Program approach to substance problems, I directed Sam to begin taking the Quick-Start nutrients to help replenish both his GABA and serotonin deficiencies. I had him begin the Power Recovery Program Detoxification nutrients as well. For the next two weeks, Sam would use these nutrients while we waited for the results of the following tests I had ordered: Amino Acid Analysis, Elemental Analysis (both Blood and Hair), Comprehensive Organix, Allergy Profile, and Fatty Acid Analysis. Because of other specific symptoms Sam had listed, I also ordered four tests I haven't mentioned previously: the Male Hormone Profile, which, as its name implies, measures levels of male hormones and in Sam's case would help determine possible causes for low sex drive; a Plasma Glucose and Insulin Levels test, for determining how well Sam's body was able to process the high levels of carbohydrates he consumed; an Adrenocortex Stress Profile test, which would measure the levels of several other key stress hormones; and an Osteoporosis Risk Evaluation, to determine Sam's potential risk for this condition, to which excessive alcohol consumption frequently contributes.

"What'd you put in those things?" Sam said with a grin when he and Doris returned for Sam's next appointment. "Those things" to which he referred were the nutritional supplements he'd been taking since his first appointment, and I took his comment to mean that he'd already noticed a difference in how he felt. He confirmed that he did feel much better, even though he didn't think any of his physical problems had had time to improve dramatically. "Mostly," he said, "I don't have the urge to drink the way I did. It's not like I've quit drinking, but I'll have two or three and stop. And it's actually a little bit easier on the days I'm not drinking. Something's going on."

Sam was right in thinking that the underlying biochemical causes and consequences of his drinking had not had time to be corrected. Despite this, the Quick-Start nutrients were having an effect. Because of them, Sam's GABA and serotonin production had almost certainly increased to the point where Sam could begin to notice a difference in the way he felt.

On this positive note, we sat down to review the results of his diagnostic tests.

One of the first things I pointed out was that Sam's Amino Acid Analysis revealed that he had very low levels of glutamine. Glutamine deficiency is implicated in many symptoms, including hypoglycemia (low blood sugar), sleep disorders, and anxiety, all of which are common among alcohol abusers. Glutamine is normally released by muscle tissue as part of the process of maintaining stable blood sugar levels. Because his glutamine levels were low, Sam craved carbohydrates, which his body used as a substitute for glutamine in attempting to stabilize his blood sugar levels. The destabilization of blood sugar levels has long been identified as a component in the craving/relapse cycle of alcoholism.

Sam's excessive carbohydrate consumption had other consequences as well. Too great an intake of carbohydrates causes an increase in the turnover and eventual depletion of serotonin, one of the brain's natural relaxing "feel-good" neurotransmitters. Since Sam's Amino Acid Analysis also confirmed what his Quick-Start questionnaire results had indicated—that he was deficient in the amino acid tryptophan, and was therefore probably unable to produce serotonin in adequate amounts—Sam, like millions of other alcohol users, relied on sugar to give him an artificial elevation of his mood. Many people who eat high-carbohydrate diets are, without knowing it, simply trying to force their brains into releasing greater amounts of serotonin, and eventually depleting the brain's supplies of this neurotransmitter. This usually happens when the nutrients needed to produce serotonin are in short supply. In this case, as in the cases of literally thousands of others I've treated, Sam had, in the process, become dependent on sweets as well as alcohol.

His glutamine deficiency also had other implications. Glutamine is one of the primary nutrients required for the production of GABA, the brain's natural valium-like stress hormone. GABA-deficient people often resort to alcohol because its GABAnergic (or GABA-enhancing) effect helps them relax and helps relieve anxiety. In addition, since the cells (called *enterocytes*) which line the intestines derive their energy from glutamine and not glucose (as most of the body's cells do), glutamine deficiency can also contribute to numerous gastrointestinal problems. Sam's Quick-Start questionnaires had identified his serotonin and GABA deficiencies, and he was already noticing the effects of glutamine, which was helping to boost his GABA production, and 5HTP, which is required for serotonin manufacture. I've found in testing thousands of patients over many years that the results of the Quick-Start questionnaires correlate very highly with the results of lab testing.

The next test I reviewed with Sam was the Glucose and Insulin Level test, which measures the levels of these substances two hours after an individual has a meal. I had ordered the test for several reasons, including Sam's being somewhat overweight, his carbohydrate consumption, and the fact that there was a history of Adult Onset Diabetes in Sam's family. I suspected that Sam was hyperinsulinemic. The test revealed that Sam's insulin levels were more than twice as high as they should have been, and that, although he was not likely to develop diabetes in the near future, he was at risk for the condition. I recommended that he immediately begin treating his hyperinsulinemia by switching to a high-protein, low-carbohydrate diet.

We moved on to Sam's Male Hormone Profile test, which indicated that his testosterone level was quite low. His low testosterone level might account in part for his lack of sex drive. Sam's Adrenocortex Stress Profile test indicated a low level of the substance DHEA, a precursor in the body's production of testosterone. I added DHEA to the list of nutrient substances in Sam's regimen. The return of Sam's sex drive, which would likely result from the increased testosterone production DHEA would stimulate, would also help to build his confidence in the treatment strategy we were pursuing. Many of the conditions now treated as "diseases" are actually only symptoms of biochemical imbalances. Correcting those imbalances with proper nutrients eliminates the disease-like conditions in a high percentage of cases.

Sam's Elemental Analysis tests showed unacceptably high levels of lead and cadmium. Sam's elevated cadmium level was probably a result of his cigarette smoking. I doubled the dosage of sulfur nutrients which Sam was already taking as part of his Detoxification protocol. Since his toxic load was significant, I also prescribed a standard heavy metal toxicity protocol, which includes various herbs, foods, and Epsom Salts baths. These rapidly and effectively chelate heavy metals. We would test the levels of these toxins and the effectiveness of Sam's treatment periodically through subsequent Urinary Elemental Analysis tests of the hair, blood, and/or urine.

The Elemental Analysis tests also revealed that Sam was deficient in zinc, vanadium, molybdenum, copper, and magnesium. Besides being cofactors in the manufacture of hundreds of proteins and enzymes in virtually every cell in our bodies, these minerals are necessary in large numbers of other biochemical processes. Magnesium alone is indispensable to more than 400 biochemical reactions that we know of. While the list of potential consequences from these deficiencies is virtually endless, I did enumerate several for Sam and Doris. Vanadium performs a function similar to that of insulin in helping maintain glucose levels, and Sam's vanadium deficiency may have contributed to his blood sugar problems. Zinc deficiencies have been associated with sexual dysfunction, prostate gland enlargement, and prostate cancer. His zinc deficiencies could certainly be a factor in Sam's sexual performance difficulties. And molybdenum is needed to increase the body's supply of sulfate, which is needed to help remove heavy metals.

Magnesium, in addition to being critical to hundreds of biochemical reactions, stabilizes all neuromuscular tissues in the body by helping to maintain the membrane "voltage," or electropotential, on the cells of these electrically charged tissues. Depleted magnesium levels cause nerve cells to fire with less-than-normal stimulation and muscles to contract more often. One of the consequences of this is that the tiny muscles that wrap around and support small blood vessels tend to squeeze down harder, causing increases in blood pressure. This is another reason why high blood pressure and other conditions in which depleted mineral levels are implicated are so often present in alcoholics.

I had ordered an Osteoporosis Risk Evaluation, a urine test which indicated that Sam was losing bone mass at an unacceptably high rate. I told him I would order further tests at a later date to see if his overall bone loss was significant enough to indicate a risk for osteoporosis. In the meantime, the mineral supplements Sam was taking as part of his Quick-Start regimen would replace his depleted supplies of essential minerals.

The Essential Fatty Acid Analysis demonstrated that Sam was deficient in Omega 3 fatty acids, which, among other things, have a powerful anti-inflammatory effect. One of the consequences of this deficiency was that Sam's body was producing arachidonic acid, a pro-inflammatory substance, in excess quantities. High levels of arachidonic acid are implicated in high blood pressure, among many other conditions. Essential fatty acids are also used in the construction and maintenance of cell membranes. Moreover, they counteract the inflammatory effects of arachidonic acid and are critical in the healing process that takes place at the cellular level in both the gastrointestinal tract and the brain. I added 3,000 mg of Omega 3 fatty acids, to be taken three times per day, to Sam's list of nutrients in the form of a product called OptiEPA, produced by Douglas Labs. This product consists of distilled, concentrated salmon oil, which is rich in Omega 3 fatty acids. Salmon oil is among the best sources for these nutrients, because salmon generally contains lower levels of mercury than many other deepsea fish, such as tuna. OptiEPA also contains very high levels of EPA, understood to be the ingredient that makes Omega 3 supplements the single most potent antidepressant we've found to date, as borne out by the published results of a number of controlled scientific studies.

Sam's Food Allergy Profile indicated, somewhat surprisingly, that, while he had some delayed sensitivities to dairy products and eggs, he was generally allergy-free. His sensitivities to eggs and dairy products were probably the result of Leaky Gut Syndrome. This condition results when damaged intestinal walls allow undigested food molecules to "leak" into the bloodstream, causing an immune system response. Immune system stress, like any other kind of stress, causes the release, and eventual depletion, of neurotransmitters and other hormones that enable us to cope, and by restricting his intake of these foods while his body healed itself, he could eliminate some of the immune system stress that might delay his recovery.

Sam's recovery was slow but steady. He found that he was able to control his drinking from the start of treatment because of the effects of the Quick-Start nutrients. Within three months, Sam was "medication-free"; that is, he had stopped taking prescription drugs altogether. To his family physician's surprise, his blood pressure remained normal and his gastrointestinal symptoms did not return. At the six-month point in his treatment, Sam was consuming only four or five drinks a week. His six-month follow-up Elemental Analysis indicated that his cadmium levels were still slightly above normal, but Sam had cut down significantly on his daily cigarette consumption and could see the day when he would also quit smoking. In the meantime, he had been eating more protein, and his carbohydrate cravings were greatly diminished. He had lost 10 pounds, and would lose an additional 25 pounds in the next six months. A follow-up insulin/glucose level test indicated he was now within normal limits, though still somewhat at the high end. Sam confessed that sexually he didn't quite feel like he was 18 again, but that at least he was starting to act his age. The amino acids and minerals in which he was deficient were also returning to normal, and I advised him to continue his present course of supplements for at least another six months.

Sam is a patient who demonstrates that so-called "alcoholics" need not engage in a constant struggle to prevent relapses. In fact, as he told me, "It was partly the fact that I didn't feel like I had to be on guard against relapsing that let me relax and get better. I can take alcohol or leave it now, but the fact that I don't have to worry if I feel like taking a drink or two is a tremendous relief. Even though I still have a drink occasionally, I'm not worried that I'm going to go overboard."

While Sam's case is typical of many people who abuse alcohol, there are also millions of people in recovery from alcohol problems who have remained sober for years but who maintain their sobriety only by extreme efforts of will. I've had hundreds of clean and sober patients tell me that even though they haven't drunk alcohol for years, they can't get through a day without thinking about taking a drink and imagining the relief they would feel. While there's often no consistent pattern to the treatments they've had—other than the fact that there's no "body" in their recovery of "mind, body, and spirit"—there is a pattern to how they describe what they're going through: They feel miserable most of the time, and they say they dream of a day when they won't have to fight with everything they have just to stay sober.

In many ways they're victims of the very treatment strategies that helped them overcome their problems. They've been led to believe that alcohol is the cause of their problems, and they've focused all of their mental, emotional, and spiritual energy on staying away from this substance. Like most alcoholics, Sam's problem was not alcohol but rather a wide array of biochemical imbalances, many of which were made worse by his alcohol and tobacco abuse. The result was a vicious cycle of worsening symptoms causing escalating substance use to mask them. But while Sam continued to use alcohol occasionally, the subject of my next case history, Sarah N., is typical of many "clean and sober" patients who come to me for treatment.

SARAH N.: CLEAN AND SOBER . . . AND STILL SUFFERING

Sarah N., a 42-year-old mother of two, came to my office to get help for her ongoing problem with alcohol. Although she also smoked cigarettes and used marijuana, she recognized that her most pressing problem was to get over her overwhelming cravings for alcohol. Unlike most alcoholic people whom I treat, however, Sarah was, as the saying goes, "in recovery." She had not had a drink for more than a year, yet, despite what doctors, counselors, and friends told her, she didn't feel better at all. On the contrary, as she put it, "I've had hangovers that weren't as bad as how I feel every day. There's nothing to hide how I feel now, and I'm here to tell you, I feel lousy. I don't remember feeling this awful before my drinking got bad, and the drinking probably didn't help, but I've got to think that the reason I let my drinking take over was because it just made me feel better."

Sarah's drinking had "taken over" about ten years ago, she explained. During the intervening years, she had been labeled a "chronic relapser" by doctors, therapists, and support group members from whom she sought help. She had undergone two three-week inpatient treatments at drug and alcohol rehabilitation facilities and several outpatient programs. She and her family had spent six months in family counseling, and she had seen three different counselors by herself. Sarah regularly attended AA meetings, even though, she told me, "A lot of the time I come out of those meetings feeling like somebody's been beating on me." She had taken several antidepressant drugs, and her doctor had prescribed Revia, a drug which may help people drink less if they relapse, but which *only works if the person taking it keeps drinking*! She had stopped taking these medications because, in her words, "They seemed to help for a while, but then they would wear off and make you feel worse." She also received Imitrex injections for her migraine headaches. Despite her substance problems, she had an excellent record at work. She and her family attended church "regularly, not every Sunday, but more often than not."

Sarah's family physician had already ordered the following diagnostic tests: CBC (Complete Blood Count), blood chemistry, T4 and TSH (thyroid studies), and a urinalysis. When the results of these tests were all well within normal limits, the doctor pronounced her "healthy as a horse." Sarah's bitter comment to me was, "I may be 'healthy as a horse,' but I doubt if he'd bet any money on me in a race."

The list of symptoms she reported to me was the same one she had given to her family physician. She had a history of intermittent heart palpitations, though several EKGs were essentially normal. She had a history of indigestion and heartburn, and she also suffered from abdominal discomfort and bloating, though tests her doctor had ordered consistently came back normal. She was a member of the "migraine-a-week club," as she put it, and she often had trouble sleeping through the night. She was frequently irritable, and, in her words, "too tired to enjoy life." Her doctor and all of her therapists had told her she was mildly depressed. She also had a skin rash that had been diagnosed as psoriasis. "And that about sums it up," she said. "I've given that list to so many people I ought to just print it out and keep copies in my purse. Not that it's done all that much good."

Sarah's Quick-Start questionnaire answers indicated that she was very probably deficient in the neurotransmitter serotonin, and she began taking the Quick-Start nutrients to help restore her serotonin production. She also began taking the Power Recovery Program Detoxification nutrients. In the meantime, I ordered the following series of diagnostic tests to pinpoint the biochemical basis of her problems: Amino Acid Analysis, Fatty Acid Analysis, Comprehensive Organix, Elemental Analysis (Blood), Allergy Profile, Comprehensive Vitamin Profile, and Comprehensive Digestive Stool Analysis. When she returned to my office two weeks later to review her test results, Sarah said, "I thought I could see some difference, but it is a little hard to tell just yet." Her tests would enable us to refine her treatment so there would be no mistaking the improvement she experienced.

Sarah's Amino Acid Analysis revealed several abnormalities. I want to review them here to help you understand how nutrient shortages are often linked together as causes of physical symptoms, and to emphasize how important and revealing these tests are for problem substance users. Sarah was deficient in the amino acids leucine and methionine. Both of these amino acids are critical in the production of enkephalins, the brain's natural painkillers, meaning that Sarah was almost certainly enkephalin-deficient. When I asked her if she had a low tolerance for pain, she replied, "How did you know?" I told her that deficiencies of leucine are a strong indicator of unusually high sensitivity to pain. Enkephalin deficiency, to which leucine deficiency contributes, is strongly implicated as a cause of alcohol cravings. In addition, methionine is required for the last stage of melatonin synthesis. Sarah's inability to synthesize enough of the sleep-inducing neurotransmitter melatonin would help explain her inability to sleep through the night.

Her Amino Acid Analysis also confirmed what her Quick-Start questionnaire had indicated: that Sarah was deficient in tryptophan. Tryptophan is required for the production of serotonin, an inhibitory (or relaxing) neurotransmitter. In addition, melatonin is made from serotonin, and Sarah's inability to produce serotonin in normal amounts further contributed to the sleep problems which were caused by already low melatonin levels. Finally, Sarah had a fairly serious taurine deficiency. Shortages of this amino acid are extremely common in people who experience heart palpitations. I directed her to add 1,500 mg of leucine, 1,500 mg of methionine, and 1,500 mg of taurine, each taken twice daily, to her Quick-Start and Detoxification nutritional supplements.

Sarah's Fatty Acid Analysis indicated she was deficient in all of the Omega 3 fatty acids. Migraine headaches have been strongly linked to shortages of Omega 3 fatty acid. Essential fatty acids are also critical for cell membrane repair, especially in the gastrointestinal tract and brain. Levels of her Omega 6 fatty acids were essentially within normal limits. I directed her to add 3,000 mg of distilled, concentrated fish oil in the form of Douglas Labs' OptiEPA, taken twice daily, to her program of supplements. We were beginning to put together a picture of the nutrient shortages which lay at the root of Sarah's symptoms. More important, we were taking the necessary steps to correct those shortages.

Sarah's Comprehensive Vitamin Profile test revealed deficiencies in vitamins B_3 and B_6, and choline. Vitamins B_3 and B_6 are indispensable in the synthesis of serotonin, and Sarah's B_6 shortage was yet another contributor to her deficiency of this critical neurotransmitter. Since she was already taking a healthy dose of B-vitamins as part of her Quick-Start regimen, there was no need for further vitamin supplements. And the lecithin she was taking as part of her Detoxification program would counteract her lack of choline.

The Elemental Analysis Blood Test revealed that Sarah was deficient in several essential minerals, including magnesium, zinc, and selenium. In addition, the level of copper in her blood was high, and her levels of tin were high enough to be considered toxic. In Sarah's high copper levels, we had found still another factor in her inability to produce serotonin, for copper toxicity inhibits the conversion of 5HTP to serotonin. Sarah's genetic risk of psoriasis (two close relatives also had the condition) was greatly increased by her zinc and selenium deficiencies, which are often implicated in skin disorders, including psoriasis. Her magnesium deficiency, along with her taurine deficiency, no doubt contributed to her heart palpitations and her anxiety. Her tin toxicity would be addressed by the Power Recovery Program Detoxification nutrients, but due to the seriousness of her toxic load, I also added a heavy metal detoxification protocol to her supplements. And I instructed her to avoid food packaged in tin cans and to use toothpaste that was tin-free (that is, which contained no stannous fluoride).

Sarah's Comprehensive Digestive Stool Analysis revealed several abnormalities. She had low levels of the digestive enzyme chymotrypsin, which breaks down proteins into smaller molecules which can be absorbed through the intestinal walls into the bloodstream. Low levels of this enzyme indicate that protein is not being completely digested, and undigested protein may be passing into the large intestine, where it can putrefy and cause irritation, gas, bloating, and the formation of toxic byproducts. Sarah also had low levels of the beneficial intestinal flora *bifidus* and *lactobacillus acidophilus.* Again, since she was already supplementing these two flora as part of her Detoxification regimen, it would very likely be only a matter of time until a healthy balance was restored.

Sarah also had very high levels of *candida albicans,* a harmful species of yeast which competes with other beneficial intestinal flora. Because her yeast overgrowth was severe, I prescribed a three-month course of the antifungal drug Lamisil, which helps treat yeast infestations outside of the intestinal tract and which is easier on the liver than most other antifungal drugs, and another antifungal, Nystatin, which treats yeast in the intestinal tract.

Finally, Sarah's Allergy Profile test revealed that she was highly allergic to wheat, peanuts, and garlic, and mildly allergic to eleven other foods. These allergies were likely caused by what is known as Leaky Gut Syndrome. This means that undigested molecules of the foods she was allergic to were slipping through the walls of the intestine into her bloodstream, where they appeared as foreign substances and caused an immune system response. She also tested highly positive to a harmful bacterium, *helicobacter pylori*. In other words, she had a chronic bacterial infection that was causing her heartburn and upset stomach. This infection, combined with her food allergies, yeast overgrowth, and digestive enzyme deficiency, contributed to her intestinal inflammation (Irritable Bowel Syndrome) and the other digestive problems she experienced.

Sarah suffered from what amounts to four kinds of stress: toxic stress, allergic stress, immune system stress, and emotional stress. They combined to rapidly deplete her levels of "stress hormones" such as serotonin and catecholamines. With her levels of these "feel-good" neurotransmitters chronically below normal, Sarah simply felt lousy all the time and didn't have the motivation or energy to get involved in positive, life-improving activities. The vicious cycle that results in cases like Sarah's is impossible to stop, and returning to health is out of the question, unless the biochemical imbalances that cause these symptoms are identified and corrected.

In Sarah's case, the correction was quite fast, taking approximately six weeks. "It's scary," she said. "I mean, I'm not sure what to do with . . . with *health*. I've never, at least not since I can remember, known what it means to be healthy. Even a little bit healthy. And this . . . "—she stepped back with a sweeping gesture—"I wouldn't believe it if somebody else told me. But it's true. And I hope that other people believe me when I tell them."

What Sarah is telling other people is not simply that she is essentially symptom-free, but that her life has changed in ways she couldn't imagine as a result. Both she and I agreed that taking care of her gastrointestinal and heavy metal problems was the key component in her rapid recovery. Within three weeks, these symptoms had all but vanished, and she really began to feel the benefits of the other nutrients she was taking. "I could sense that they were making a difference from the start," she said, "but when my stomach and intestinal problems began to disappear, they really kicked in. It was like my body was, pardon the language, *kickin' butt* on all those conditions now that it had what it needed. My outlook brightened, my skin cleared up, I began to sleep through the night, my head didn't hurt anymore, I got my energy back . . . you name it, it got better. And I know it's going to stay that way."

CONCLUSION

Alcohol problems, in addition to being among the most pervasive of all substance disorders, are also associated with the broadest array of secondary biochemical conditions. Gastrointestinal problems are endemic among heavy alcohol users, and they are often compounded by the fact that most physicians do not know how to treat them except by masking the symptoms with drugs. From migraine headaches to sleep disorders to osteoporosis, heavy alcohol users often suffer a truly diverse and extraordinary array of cascade effect symptoms. Traditional approaches to these conditions often rely on everything from "sleeping pills" to painkillers, and in doing so avoid treating the true causes. In addition, mood disorders, from depression to anxiety to bipolar illness, which are extremely common among those who abuse alcohol, are often exacerbated by traditional medical and psychiatric treatments, in which powerful psychotropic substances are added to the toxic load and neurotransmitter deficiencies to which alcohol contributes.

As with virtually all cases of substance abuse, excessive alcohol use is usually one of a set of biochemically caused conditions which are often simply misdiagnosed and incorrectly treated. Using biochemical testing as the basis for rebalancing biochemistry, alcohol abusers now have a proven, science-based method for getting to the root of their problems and correcting them. The results, as you can see, include nothing less than the renewed hope for living a healthy life.

12

Overcoming the Consequences of Cocaine and Amphetamine Abuse

In this chapter I'll deal with the effects of the long-term use of cocaine, with some mention of the abuse of prescription stimulants, including Ritalin and amphetamines. Cocaine and Ritalin are classed among the most addictive substances available. Brain imagery studies have shown that both substances disrupt the neurotransmitter dopamine in identical ways, and excessive use of either Ritalin or cocaine can lead to the same cascade effect symptoms.

In Chapter 16, I'll deal with a special case of prescription stimulant use by children when I focus my attention on the abuse of the drug Ritalin, a cocaine-like drug which is indiscriminately used to treat millions of children diagnosed with Attention Deficit Disorder (ADD) and Attention Deficit/Hyperactivity Disorder (ADHD). In that chapter I'll concentrate on how we can avoid exposing children to the potential for brain damage and addiction which prescription psychotropic drugs can cause, and on the fact that there are safe, effective ways to eliminate the symptoms for which they are prescribed by addressing the underlying biochemical causes. But in this chapter, as you'll see in the following case history, both Mark and Lena, like millions of other stimulant abusers, used Ritalin and amphetamines when they were unable to obtain cocaine. As you'll also see, overcoming the abuse of stimulants is often a fairly straightforward matter, and the outcomes are overwhelmingly positive for those using the Power Recovery Program protocols.

CASCADE EFFECT CONDITIONS
RESULTING FROM ACUTE STIMULANT ABUSE

Many of the long-term cascade effect symptoms of stimulant abuse—including high blood pressure and the risk of heart attack-are familiar to most people. Below, a number of these conditions are discussed.

Cocaine and amphetamines both cause vasoconstriction (tightening of the muscles around the blood vessels throughout the body). When either is ingested by sniffing through the nose, the mucous membranes in the nose can erode and die. After cocaine use, reflex vasodilation (loosening of the muscles around the blood vessels in the nose) can occur, causing fluid to leak out into the nasal cavity and resulting in what appears to be a "runny nose." This condition is referred to as *chronic rhinitis* and is considered a cascade effect symptom of stimulant abuse.

Bronchitis is another condition that can result from stimulant use. When cocaine is smoked in the form of "crack," the toxins taken into the lungs irritate the cells and connective tissue of the tiny air pockets that line the interior of the lungs. The resulting damage can cause a chronic cough and make crack smokers susceptible to upper respiratory infections.

Anxiety and panic attacks can result from stimulant use, because receptors for excitatory neurotransmitters are overstimulated. Stimulant drugs, because they take the place of catecholamines, our excitatory neurotransmitters, can eventually dramatically decrease the brain's ability to produce excitatory neurotransmitters, often resulting in serious *mood disorders,* especially depression.

We experience hunger as an unpleasant sensation partly because the falling levels of amino acids in our blood that occur when we have not eaten for several hours reduce the brain's ability to produce adequate amounts of excitatory neurotransmitters. Stimulants occupy catecholamine receptors in the brain, sending a false signal that the need for food has been satisfied. Because of this, chronic stimulant abusers frequently go for long periods of time, even days, without eating, and this behavior, over time, causes *malnutrition.*

Like nicotine, stimulant drugs affect catecholamine receptors in the muscles of the heart, causing the heart to become overstimulated and irritated. If the irritation is severe enough, *heart arrhythmia* or *palpitations* can result. This condition can result in an increase in the risk of heart attacks in people who use stimulants.

Chest pain can have many and varied causes, including irritation of the esophagus, lungs, or heart muscle, all of which can be made worse by the use of stimulants. Even experienced doctors often have difficulty determining the precise cause of chest pain, and anyone experiencing this symptom should seek immediate medical help.

The overstimulation of excitatory neurotransmitter receptors caused by stimulants can lead to difficulty falling or staying asleep. So *sleep disorders* are yet another cascade effect symptom of stimulant use.

Chronic abuse of stimulants exhausts the brain's ability to produce relaxing neurotransmitters, which are in high demand when stimulants are used. Therefore, such abuse often markedly increases the risk of *violent and other criminal/psychotic behavior* which is normally regulated by relaxing neurotransmitters. This is why stimulant use is frequently associated with bizarre and unpredictable natures.

These conditions are discussed in more detail in the following case histories. I want to emphasize that these case histories are meant to provide you with a *model* for seeking treatment and correcting any cascade effect symptoms your stimulant abuse may have caused. These secondary conditions, many of which can become very serious if left uncorrected, develop as a result of many factors, including genetics, stress levels, diet, and exposure to toxins. The best way to determine the precise biochemical causes of cascade effect symptoms is to have biochemical testing done by a qualified lab.

MARK AND LENA W.: WHEN GO-GETTERS GET OUT OF CONTROL

The first words out of Mark's mouth when he and his wife, Lena, walked into my office for their initial appointment were, "Look, I'm really sorry about . . . well, about the way we look, I guess is what I'm trying to say. It sounds kind of hollow, but don't judge us by appearances." Mark and Lena were in crisis. They had called my office earlier in the day, and, after talking to Mark on the phone, I arranged to see him and his wife at 6:00 pm, after normal office hours. Their appearance was indeed unusual. Both of them wore what appeared to be expensive clothes. Mark, I later learned, was wearing a Hugo Boss suit; Lena had on what could only be described as a "classy" navy-blue linen blazer and slacks outfit. The reason for Mark's apology was that it looked as though both of them had just returned from a week camping out and had forgotten to take a change of clothes with them. And as it turned out, Mark's apology notwithstanding, their clothes *were* a pretty good way to judge the shape they were in.

"I guess it started about a year, year and a half ago," Mark said, looking at Lena. She nodded. "I mean, is this what you need to know? How we got into this shape?" I told him I had a pretty good idea of what had been going on, but that I wanted to hear the story from him and Lena. They shared in the telling of their story. They had met at the real estate office where Mark was a top salesman when Lena, who had her own bookkeeping and accounting business, took on the company as a client. They were immediately attracted to each other and began dating within a few days of their first meeting.

"I think the attraction was so strong because we have a lot in common," Lena told me. "We're both real go-getters. We both like to work hard. We just clicked." They were married less than four months after they met, and in the two years following their wedding, Mark rose to the top of the agency's sales force. Lena allowed her business to level off somewhat, keeping five of her best clients. During this time, they entertained often. "If there was a pattern," Mark explained, "I guess you could say it consisted of plenty of drinking, followed by plenty of hangovers. But I guess the *problem*, well, just kind of snuck up on us," Mark went on. "The cocaine, I mean." They had stayed later than usual at a party given by one of their friends, and, at about 2 am, the host began to lay out lines of cocaine for Mark and Lena and one other couple. "It just livened things up so much, well, I couldn't believe it," Lena went on. "We laughed and talked, and the next thing we knew the sun was coming up. We did not want to go home, let me tell you. We did not want that party to end. I guess you could say we did everything we could to make sure it didn't. For about a year and a half."

Mark was making plenty of money, so, in Lena's words, "We figured, nothing to worry about, right? We had it, why not spend it?" Their spending, along with their cocaine habits, quickly went out of control. Within less than four months they found they were getting behind in their bills. Four months after that, they began looking for ways to make extra money just to support their habits. "Working harder was not one of options we explored," Lena explained.

"I made almost $350,000.00 in commissions in my best year," Mark said. "It just didn't make sense that we could spend it all." They had been living well, and their everyday living expenses were high, but when they tried to sit down and calculate what they were spending on drugs, they couldn't quite believe it. "We came up with somewhere around $1,000 a day," Lena said. "How we could have been spending that much I still can't tell you, and I'm an accountant. But we were. That much and more."

Mark's professional performance slipped dramatically. Most of the time he was moody and hard to get along with. He used the term "strung out," which I've heard from many of my patients, to describe his condition. As time went on, he began to miss appointments with prospective clients. He hadn't closed a sale in more than two months. Only the fact that he'd recently been a top performer kept his boss from dismissing him.

While cocaine was their drug of choice, and while they preferred to snort powdered cocaine, two things happened fairly quickly. First, they discovered that Ritalin and amphetamines were very easy to obtain, and they began using them instead of cocaine when their regular supplier was out. Both of them found Ritalin to be virtually "as good as cocaine." Second, they discovered "crack." This form of cocaine, which comes in "rock" form and is smoked rather than sniffed, causes a much more intense, though shorter-lived, "high" than powdered cocaine. It also causes cravings which are far more intense than those for powdered cocaine, which is itself capable of causing very serious cravings.

Their habits had reached, in Mark's words, "some sort of limit." He went on to explain: "Even if we hadn't run out of money, we've just run out of time and out of the physical resources to recover. We've been using literally every day for six months, and we just can't do it anymore. We hit the wall." Because they both worked out of offices in their home, they had to a great extent been able to conceal their drug use. But both agreed that at some point it must have become fairly obvious to those around them that they were using drugs heavily. In addition to the other problems caused by their drug use, one of the side effects especially associated with amphetamines was that both were becoming very paranoid.

As it turned out, their paranoia was not totally without justification. About three months before they first came to see me, their financial situation had gotten so serious that they had to look for a way to make money quickly. It was partly the very real fear that the money-making strategy they finally came up with might land Lena in jail which had finally brought them to my office. For the past two and a half months, Lena had been embezzling money from the real estate office where Mark worked. "Of course we knew it was illegal," she said. "On some level, we were aware of the risks. God, living every day with the fear of being caught . . . ." Lena's voice trailed off. I didn't need to point out to them that the increased stress associated with their embezzlement scheme only intensified their need for cocaine.

While Mark's primary substances of abuse were stimulants, Lena's use of stimulants was compounded by the fact that she also took the anti-depressant drug Paxil. She had had panic attacks in the past, and she frequently called her doctor for refills of the drug, which he was always ready to prescribe.

They were impatient for some sort of quick resolution I might provide for them, but they did cooperate by filling out questionnaires after I had briefly explained my approach to treating substance problems. Lena's Quick-Start questionnaire answers indicated that she was deficient in both tyrosine and serotonin, which her pattern of drug use clearly suggested. Mark's questionnaire answers indicated a tyrosine deficiency. I prescribed double doses of the Quick-Start nutrients, along with the normal dose of Detoxification nutrients appropriate for both of them, and, considering the condition they were in, gave them their first two doses of the Quick-Start nutrients right in my office. We then went on to discuss further treatment.

I recommended that both of them check into a detoxification facility so that they could receive the intensive inpatient treatment they needed. While Mark rejected the idea, Lena agreed to it. Mark argued that he needed to quit using drugs and get back to work so he could try to get them back on track financially. For Lena, checking into a rehabilitation hospital made sense. The real estate agency had called for an audit of its finances, and Lena was certain her embezzlement scheme would be discovered. In addition to offering her the opportunity to stop using drugs, a stay in the hospital would indicate that she was serious about recovery, which, she reasoned, would help in any legal defense they had to mount. Both were determined to pay back the money they had stolen, and they were ready to do what had to be done to convince others of their sincerity.

Mark was insistent that he could stop using stimulants, and I, of course, couldn't order him to enter a drug rehabilitation facility. But I did get him to agree to undergo frequent urine tests to confirm that he was abstaining from drug use. He also agreed to enter an intensive outpatient therapy program, which included group therapy sessions four times per week and daily attendance at AA meetings. Mark also agreed to attend a family therapy group meeting at the detoxification facility where Lena was a patient.

In telling you about their treatment, and how they were able to recover from a dire situation, I'm going to focus on two things: how they corrected the biochemical imbalances that led them to their substance abuse, and how they made what I call a spiritual discovery about themselves and each other. First let me talk about their treatment. Both suffered from chronic rhinitis ("runny nose") because they snorted cocaine, and chronic bronchitis from smoking crack. Both Mark and Lena also had heart palpitations, but Mark didn't take them seriously. Mark had no other significant symptoms. Lena confessed that, in addition to experiencing panic attacks (which were becoming more difficult to control as their situation became more desperate), she had recently been contemplating suicide. While she knew in her heart that she wanted to live, she was fearful that she might actually commit suicide when she was under the influence of drugs.

While Lena would receive a full battery of tests as part of her inpatient treatment, I ordered several tests for Mark through his primary care physician. These included an EKG, CBC (Complete Blood Count), and blood chemistries. I also ordered Amino Acid Analysis and Elemental Analysis tests for both Mark and Lena. Mark and Lena had health insurance through a private company, and their coverage was excellent.

Three days later, when the results of his EKG came across my desk, I called Mark on the phone immediately with the news that the test showed "Q waves" in the inferior leads, an indication that he might have suffered a heart attack at some time in the past, though probably not within the past several weeks. Mark confirmed on the phone that he had suffered chest pains on several occasions, but that he thought they were the result of bronchial irritation from smoking crack. I immediately referred him to a cardiologist, who ordered a catheterization, which confirmed that Mark had indeed had a heart attack but that the area on the left lower side of his heart was stable and he suffered no arterial blockage. This indicated that the heart attack was very likely a result of *vasospasm* (sudden constriction or cramping of a blood vessel) caused by cocaine use. Mark's cardiologist advised him that, since he had suffered no significant damage from his heart attack, the main thing he needed to do to avoid further complications was to refrain from abusing stimulants. This certainly helped fuel Mark's drive to become substance-free.

Although excessive use of stimulants can be extremely dangerous, in fact, cocaine abuse is in many ways one of the most treatable of substance problems. Given the condition in which many cocaine and amphetamine abusers come to me for treatment, however, it's not something I bring up early in their treatment. Both Mark and Lena experienced what Lena called "miraculous" reductions in their drug cravings virtually immediately upon beginning the Power Recovery Program Quick-Start nutrients. So rapidly did their Quick-Start nutrients "kick in," in fact, that I could see small changes in their behavior and demeanor even before they left my office that first evening. I've observed this kind of dramatic reduction of cravings and mood swings in hundreds upon hundreds of cocaine and amphetamine abusers. Both Mark and Lena agreed that it was one of the keys to their recoveries. Despite the fact that both were clearly susceptible to immediately relapsing, the early indications that they were experiencing positive effects from their nutrients gave me confidence that they would be able to make it through that first night without having to use any drugs.

Lena's supervising physician and I talked often during her recovery at the detoxification facility. He agreed to be present when we reviewed her biochemical tests, and he supported her use of nutrients as part of her therapy. I had ordered Amino Acid Analysis and Elemental Analysis tests for Lena, and the results indicated deficiencies of the amino acids methionine, cysteine, and tryptophan, with a slight tyrosine deficiency. Methionine is required for the production of the sleep-inducing neurotransmitter melatonin, and it is also necessary for the production of enkephalins. Although her essential mineral levels were within normal limits, Lena had slightly elevated levels of lead and cadmium. The latter was a result of her having been a cigarette smoker for about ten years, until she quit more than five years ago. The Power Recovery Program Detoxification nutrients would bring her lead and cadmium levels down to normal within a matter of months, and I added 1,500 mg of both methionine and cysteine, taken three times per day, to Lena's nutritional supplement protocol.

Within a matter of less than two weeks, when Mark next came to my office to review his biochemical tests, I saw a changed man. I hesitate to use the word "chastened," but something in his attitude and demeanor told me he was taking a difficult lesson to heart (double meaning intended) and would emerge from his experience a stronger person. His blood chemistries and CBC (Complete Blood Count) had all come back within normal limits. His Amino Acid Analysis revealed that, in addition to the tyrosine deficiency predicted by his Quick-Start questionnaire results, he was deficient in taurine, phenylalanine, and cysteine. His Elemental Analysis test revealed deficiencies in the essential minerals magnesium, potassium, and selenium. Both magnesium and potassium are essential for maintaining good heart and brain health, and selenium deficiencies are often associated with skin disorders.

When both Mark and Lena came into my office three months after they had first been there, I was given some insight into the nature of the change Mark had undergone. Even though he himself was still in crisis during the first weeks of his recovery, he had visited Lena in the hospital every day. He cried unashamedly when he explained that he suddenly realized how important Lena was to him. "She looked so forlorn in that hospital. I realized that, even though we were both responsible for our actions, by behaving the way *I* did I put the person I loved more than anyone in the world in jeopardy. I could have stood up at any time and said, 'Let's put a stop to this today,' but I didn't. But I'm doing that now. I'm putting a stop to it. I know she is, too."

For Mark and Lena, the discovery that each of them had something—perhaps I should say *someone*—to live for besides the pursuit of a good party was one of the keys to their recovery. Mark's turnaround was very fast. His body responded immediately to the Power Recovery Program nutritional supplements, and he was quick to say that the realization of how much Lena meant to him could not have happened unless he had achieved the physical results he did from the nutrients. Lena spent only twelve days of her projected three-week stay in the hospital. She felt that she had reached a point of diminishing returns and that she'd actually be able to complete her recovery better outside the hospital. By that time I had no qualms about seeing her released. She, too, had made great strides toward recovery, and she said that more than anything she wanted to be with Mark. And thanks to the extra dopamine their brains were now producing, they both rekindled the simple joy of being in love in an authentic and life-affirming way.

I've learned something watching so many of my patients rebuild their lives: It never hurts to have fate on your side. And as fate would have it, Mark's boss was a recovering alcoholic. He had been clean and sober for more than fifteen years, and when Mark and Lena approached him about what they had done, he was very understanding. He himself had built his agency from the ground up only after a very difficult recovery, and he was willing to work with Mark and Lena as they made restitution of the money they had stolen. In him, Mark and Lena found an ally. "We're even talking to him about taking nutrients," Mark said, "but he may be harder to convince than we were." He added quickly, "Not that that's necessarily a bad thing, you understand."

CONCLUSION

Although cocaine and amphetamine abuse can quickly escalate to crisis proportions, I want to reiterate that stopping the use of these substances is often a fairly straightforward proposition. Although cocaine dramatically disrupts the neurotransmitter dopamine, large doses of tyrosine can quickly—often within hours—begin to restore the nutrients necessary to correct the disruption. Many cocaine and amphetamine users report immediate noticeable reductions in their cravings for these substances. They also report that as long as they continue to supplement with tyrosine and the other Quick-Start nutrients, they don't experience the low-energy "crash" or depression that so often accompanies stimulant recovery for the first several months. As one of my patients put it, "The nutrients take the fear out of stopping. I was actually afraid of what might happen if I quit, afraid of facing those cravings and that awful depression. But there's no need to feel that way. Not if you're taking the nutrients."

I want to make it clear, however, that even though nutrients can take the fear out of quitting, nutrients do *not* get you "high" the way drugs do. You should not think that somehow, by taking nutrients that reduce or eliminate your stimulant cravings, you will find yourself walking around feeling like you do when you use cocaine. That's obviously not a realistic expectation, and it's not something I would ever mislead my patients into believing.

Catecholamine restoration brings other benefits besides avoidance of the difficult symptoms that can accompany withdrawal from cocaine abuse. These benefits include being able to think clearly, not being physically dependent on a substance, knowing you're not threatening your health and your family's welfare, and being able to pursue the activities which will truly enable you to achieve personal and professional satisfaction instead of constantly focusing on obtaining your substance of abuse. And my take on that goes something like this: Even if what I'm describing doesn't meet your criteria for being "high," it's still an awfully good outcome.

13

Overcoming the Consequences of Abusing Opiates and Painkillers

Morphine, the psychotropic substance in opium poppies, has been the most effective painkiller available to physicians since the mid-nineteenth century, when the invention of the hypodermic needle provided a way to administer the substance to patients. Two other substances, heroin and opium, which are also derived from opium poppies, have been ingested by smoking or in liquid form for an even longer time by those seeking the escape into the euphoria and freedom from pain that they provide. Today a number of substances, from prescription painkillers such as Darvon to heroin substitutes such as methadone, are widely used in both medical treatment and "recreationally."

All of these substances act directly on receptors for endorphins and enkephalins, the brain's natural painkilling neurotransmitters. I've outlined how and why they work in Chapter 3, and I won't spend a great deal of time in review here. I will emphasize, however, that all of these substances are potentially highly addictive and that the recent rise in their use by young people—labeled "heroin chic" by print and electronic journalists always happy to oblige with publicity for the latest cultural trend—represents a dangerous though not terribly widespread phenomenon. The case history I'll be starting with in this chapter is, in fact, virtually a textbook illustration of the consequences of heroin use among young men and women. The second case history highlights a problem—physician shopping, or working with more than one physician to prescribe psychotropic substances—that has become increasingly serious as people tend increasingly to abuse prescription drugs.

CASCADE EFFECT CONDITIONS
RESULTING FROM OPIATE ABUSE

Unlike those of many substances, the long-term cascade effect symptoms of opiate abuse—including malnutrition and chronic pain—are not familiar to most people. Below is a discussion of a number of these conditions:

We experience hunger as an unpleasant sensation partly because the falling levels of amino acids in our blood that occur when we have not eaten for several hours prevent the brain from producing adequate amounts of neurotransmitters such as endorphins and enkephalins (the brain's natural painkilling neurotransmitters). Opiates artificially stimulate endorphin/enkephalin receptors in the brain, sending the false signal that there are plenty of endorphins and enkephalins and that the brain's requirements for protein are satisfied. This has the effect of "short-circuiting" hunger, making the opioid user unaware of the fact that she needs to eat. If this occurs frequently over time, a condition of general *malnutrition* (common in opioid abusers) can result.

Chronic pain is another cascade effect symptom of opiate abuse. By occupying endorphin and enkephalin receptors in the brain, opioid drugs cause a down-regulation (or reduction) in the normal production of the body's natural painkilling neurotransmitters to compensate for the over-abundance of artificial opioids. After long-term use, when the drug is not present, even minor physical or emotional pain can be perceived as very severe, because the brain is relatively incapable of producing endorphins and enkephalins to counteract it.

Amino acid deficiencies are a problem for many who abuse opiates. Endorphins and enkephalins are made from several amino acids (including tyrosine, glycine, phenylalanine, leucine, and methionine) that are commonly deficient in opiate abusers. These deficiencies cause the brain's ability to produce them to be compromised, which can cause opiate cravings. The use of opiates, in turn, causes malnutrition, which worsens the nutrient shortage and causes a "vicious cycle" of substance craving, substance use, and worsened nutrient shortage.

These conditions are discussed in more detail in the following case histories. I want to emphasize that these case histories are meant to provide you with a *model* for seeking treatment and correcting any cascade effect symptoms your opiate abuse may have caused. These secondary conditions, many of which can become very serious if left uncorrected, develop as a result of many factors, including genetics, stress levels, diet, and exposure to toxins. The best way to determine the precise biochemical causes of cascade effect symptoms is to have biochemical testing done by a qualified laboratory.

TONY P.: RIDIN' THE WAVE

On his first visit to my office, 24-year-old Tony P. was, in his words, "a little strung out." Zero Point Energy, the rock band for which Tony played lead guitar, had just come off a two-and-a-half month tour of the East Coast in support of their recently released CD. In larger cities, they had been relegated to opening for better known bands, but they received top billing in at least a dozen smaller venues. They had played more than fifty dates in seventy days, and, as Tony put it, "the road just caught up with me." I got the distinct impression that he viewed me as something like a medic in a war zone. He didn't come out and say, "You've got to get me patched up so I can get back out there," but that message came through loud and clear, at least initially.

"The road," as Tony described it, was an ongoing party of epic proportions. "The problem is," he explained, "that the people who come out to hear us, well, it's a big party night for them, but then they can go home and rest up till the next weekend or till the next band comes through. But we don't have five or six days off to recover. It's our job not to disappoint them. We've got to party as hard as we can every night. There's no letup for us. And there's only one way to keep up the pace: drugs."

Tony had sampled a large variety of psychotropic substances, from cocaine and amphetamines to alcohol to marijuana, but, as he put it, "For me, it always kept coming back to heroin." Early in the tour he'd tried the drug for the first time, sniffing it in powder form. For him, it made all the pressure of being on tour "just disappear, at least for a couple of hours." Within a few weeks, he was using heroin almost every day. At first he avoided it before performances, using it only to "party" with after a show. But as the tour ground on, he'd begun to use heroin shortly after he woke up, often staying high on the drug throughout the day and evening. He wasn't worried, he said, "because I was just snorting. You know, I mean, how serious could it be?"

When heroin wasn't available, he used alcohol heavily to help him get through the day without his drug of choice. About three weeks before the end of the tour, he'd met a girl who began traveling with him. Following her lead, he began to "shoot up," that is, to inject heroin directly into his bloodstream. Re-experiencing the intense euphoria that came from injecting the drug quickly became the focus of his life. "It was a good thing I'd played our songs about a thousand times, because I wasn't paying much attention and my memory was messed up. I was going through the motions on stage. Couldn't wait to get to the party."

The party stopped abruptly. The band's drummer was injured in an auto accident, and all the dates of the final three weeks of the tour were canceled. Tony's new girlfriend disappeared, in his words, "within hours." Suddenly Tony was forced to figure out what he was going to do with a long string of empty days ahead of him. "It was like I had to, you know, *decompress* or something. All of that intense energy and pressure that keeps driving you forward . . . it just wasn't there. I'd been ridin' the wave, and all of a sudden, dead calm."

Tony was a very bright young man, and he became immediately fascinated when I began to explain to him how heroin achieved its effects by disrupting endorphins and enkephalins, the brain's natural painkilling neurotransmitters. As I explained the role of nutrition in maintaining biochemical balance, he chuckled. "Nutrition? What's that? I'm sorry, I don't mean to be a wise guy, but it's almost like I can't relate to what you're talking about. There's plenty of food on the road, but I wouldn't begin to know what I should eat. I haven't eaten a vegetable for years. That probably tells you something."

Tony's physical condition reflected the serious deficiencies in his diet. He was 6 feet tall and weighed 149 pounds, but, unlike many slender people, he had very little lean muscle mass. Otherwise his physical exam results were normal. Both of Tony's problems, with nutrition and with drug use, went back at least ten years. He was "hangin' out, gettin' high" on a regular basis by the time he was 14 years old. By age 16, he was stopping by his parents' home "maybe two or three times a week." He spent most of his time at a dilapidated house rented by one of the members of the band for whom he "ran errands and just generally did what needed to be done, you know, helping them move equipment and set up, that kind of stuff." He had quit school and was learning how to play guitar. He recalled that nobody had any money for food, but that there always seemed to be beer and pot around.

This type of existence had characterized Tony's lifestyle until a few years ago when he and another friend formed Zero Point Energy and that band began to gain a local following. "After that," he said, "what changed was not the lifestyle itself, but the fact that there was more of it. More money, more drugs, that kind of thing." He now wondered openly if he could walk away from that life. He also wondered if he could stay in it without getting overwhelmed by drugs. Since he was not committed to rehearsals or performances for at least a couple of months, he thought he'd try to, in his words, "at least clean up my act some."

I ordered the following tests for Tony: Amino Acid Analysis, Elemental Analysis, Essential Fatty Acid Analysis, Allergy Profile, Complete Blood Count, and blood chemistries. Tony had no health insurance, but, having money in the bank as a result of his band's recent successes, he willingly paid for the tests out of pocket. While we waited for the results of his tests, Tony would be taking the Power Recovery Program Detoxification nutrients and the Quick-Start nutrients to correct enkephalin/endorphin deficiencies.

I had prescribed medication, including Motrin for pain, Clonidine for anxiety, and Lomotil for diarrhea, to help Tony through what I explained to him would be a difficult withdrawal period, although one which would very likely not pose medical problems. By the time he had stopped using heroin for three days, he was suffering from withdrawal symptoms, including achiness, stomach pain, and headaches, which made him very uncomfortable. Drinking alcohol helped reduce his symptoms, but he agreed that he would try to continue to refrain from using heroin and stop drinking as his body detoxified and the medication began to take effect. I explained that he would soon begin to re-establish baseline nutrient levels that would make him feel better and make him less susceptible to relapsing.

Although I recommended that Tony check into a detoxification facility, he assured me that he had the necessary support system to ensure that he could succeed in stopping his heroin use. He was staying with another band member who had a stable marriage and who was committed to helping Tony kick his habit.

Two weeks later, when Tony returned to review his test results, he said that his acute withdrawal symptoms were not nearly as bad as they

had been, but he nonetheless described himself as "in the doldrums." I
explained that I wasn't surprised, given the duration and intensity of the
"party" he'd been living, but I quickly qualified that statement. Recovering from a party wasn't the only thing making Tony miserable. While his
Allergy Profile showed no problems, and while his blood tests were normal, Tony was deficient in every one of the amino acids and almost every
essential mineral tested for. He was also very deficient in both Omega 3
and Omega 6 essential fatty acids. With typical sardonic humor, he said,
"That's gotta be some kind of record, right?"

"Other than the fact that you've been running on empty, probably for
years, you're not in bad shape," I told him. To my surprise, he caught the
Jackson Browne reference I'd slipped in. I continued, telling him, "Given
your history, you're probably going to hate me for this, but you've got to
start eating. A lot. Three meals a day, at least, and protein shakes, as
many as you want." In addition to his Quick-Start and Detoxification
nutrients, I added 2,000 mg of the amino acids tyrosine and glutamine,
taken three times per day, and 200 mg of 5HTP, also taken three times per
day. I also prescribed 3,000 mg of the essential fatty acid supplement
Super EPA 500, by Douglas Labs (which would provide Omega 3 fatty
acids), to be taken three times per day, and one 500 mg capsule of borage
oil (for Omega 6 fatty acids), to be taken once per day. And I prescribed
mixed digestive enzymes to help his body process the significant increases in nutrients.

"That's it?" he asked skeptically. "That's it," I said. "It's not necessarily complicated, but it is required. If you give your body what it needs,
your body will give you what you need. Within limits, of course. You
can't hammer yourself indefinitely with drugs and alcohol, even if you
are eating right. I know that this might sound unbelievable, but I think
you'll find that simply taking supplements and eating enough to keep
your nutrient levels up will make it so you don't need to do that anymore. Try it and see for yourself."

Tony did try it. And he shared his outcome with me. Tony and I
developed something akin to a friendship as we got to know each other,
and when he was no longer a "patient," he'd call me on the phone occasionally just to talk. Something he said during one of our many informal
conversations was very gratifying to me: "You know, one of the things I
appreciate is that you never told me I had to stop completely or I'd die,

you never tried to scare me into getting clean, and as a result, I've always been honest with you. I still may not be a poster boy for a drug-free society, but I'm not going to kill myself, either. And I've managed to bring your message, if that's what you'd call it, to a lot of other people."

The recovery behind those words involved Tony's gradually restoring his baseline levels of amino acids, minerals, and essential fatty acids to within normal ranges. As he started to put on weight, he decided to "go to the gym." By the time Zero Point Energy began rehearsing again more than three months later, Tony had discovered that, in fact, he probably didn't need drugs to keep ahead of "the road." Although he didn't quit using substances altogether, he reported that his drug use had become "so casual you'd have to look hard to know that I indulged at all," and that he'd stopped using heroin completely. The important thing, as Tony discovered, was that because of the biochemical changes he'd brought about, he was in control in a way he'd never been before.

While it's easy to identify the obvious cases of opiate abuse such as Tony's, the problem is by no means limited to young people. Nor is it limited to "street" drugs such as heroin. Opiates come in many forms, and by far the majority of them are, unlike heroin, perfectly legal and used for the legitimate medical purpose of helping people deal with pain. But like heroin, prescription painkilling drugs are potentially highly addictive, and their abuse can have consequences as damaging as that of heroin.

BETH C.: LET THE SELLER BEWARE

Beth C. was a successful businessperson who liked to "shop." She shopped everything she bought, both as Purchasing Director for her employer, a large manufacturing company, and as a consumer. Among other things, Beth shopped doctors. In fact, at one time she had six primary care physicians simultaneously. She also occasionally saw a chiropractor, an acupuncturist, and a massage therapist.

At age 40, Beth had been riding horses for more than twenty years. She had had "three or four minor spills" during her first several years of riding, and was bothered by chronic joint and muscle pain. She attributed her pain to injuries, which she had ignored at the time they occurred, suffered in those early falls. More recently, however, she had suffered a more serious injury, rupturing three discs in her back when she fell from one of the three horses she owned. Although she was hospitalized in traction for two weeks as she recovered from the fall, she adamantly refused to consider surgery.

While she claimed she wanted to be "conservative" in her approach to treating the injury, there was an ulterior motive in her refusing to submit to surgery. For several years before her fall, Beth had been developing a reliance on painkilling drugs which, after her most recent injury, threatened to blossom into a full-blown addiction. Her propensity to shop doctors, while it appeared to demonstrate that she was a careful consumer, was actually a tactic which insured that she would always have a ready supply of Darvon, codeine, or hydrocodone, the substances she abused. She would never have to "burn out" any of her sources for the drugs, because she visited each of her doctors only every three or four months.

Her strategy had been uncovered during her hospital stay when the company physician, who was familiar with Beth's medical history, noticed discrepancies in the primary care physician she listed upon admission to the hospital and the one listed on her company medical records. When he followed up with the doctors, he discovered that Beth had been seeing both of them for treatment of chronic pain and that both had prescribed painkillers. In one instance, her appointments with the two doctors were less than three weeks apart from each other. He immediately suspected that Beth was "playing both ends from the middle," and he discussed his suspicions with her just before she checked out of the hospital. She admitted that she had a substance problem.

The company doctor, who was familiar with my approach to treating substance abuse, recommended that Beth make an appointment with me immediately, and that she use the remaining recovery time, before she returned to work, to begin to deal with her problem. Beth told me that, while she was initially "frightened" that she might be somehow punished for what she'd done, she was also relieved that she'd been "caught." The company doctor assured her that her medical history would remain confidential. His primary concern was that she seek assistance for her substance problem. She agreed to follow his recommendation.

Beth's company-paid insurance was among the best available, and the tests I ordered, including an Elemental Analysis, an Amino Acid Analysis, an Essential Fatty Acid Analysis (all from blood samples), and a Comprehensive Organix, were paid for by the insurance company. I explained the strategy that I would recommend for her gradual withdrawal from opiates. I also prescribed the Power Recovery Program enkephalin/ endorphin Quick-Start nutrients and the Detoxification nutrients, which she would take while we awaited her test results. I knew that it was critical that Beth get "natural" relief from pain in order to prevent her from returning to the use of prescription painkillers. I therefore prescribed several other nutrients that would help her begin the process of repairing damaged cartilage and help to reduce her pain. These substances included glucosamine sulfate, chondroitin sulfate, and bromelain. I explained that much of the cartilage in the body receives its nutrient supply not from the blood (as with other tissues), but from the fluids that bathe the cartilage. I prescribed physical therapy, including stretching, swimming, and yoga, to help stimulate the delivery of nutrients to the chondrocytes, the cells that carry out cartilage repair.

Part of her recovery strategy would include, I told her, my notifying the physicians from whom she had sought treatment that she was in recovery and that they were not to prescribe painkillers for her. Although this method is, of course, not foolproof, it would serve to lessen her temptation to revert to her previous behavior.

Because she had a long-term problem with painkillers, I chose a conservative withdrawal strategy which included close medical supervision. Opioid withdrawal can be very difficult under the best of circumstances, and, in this case, the non-narcotic drug Clonidine, administered initially in pill form and subsequently through a patch, would help ease her through the initial weeks. Clonidine would help alleviate many of the symptoms associated with withdrawal from opioids. She would withdraw on an outpatient basis under the close supervision of a nurse, who would visit her daily and who would make sure that she tapered her opioid use gradually. In this case, tapering meant reducing her daily doses by 20 to 25 percent each week. While I would normally strongly recommend that she withdraw in a detoxification facility, Beth would also be receiving strong support from her husband, and I felt that she would be able to succeed on an outpatient basis.

Beth's biochemical test results indicated widespread deficiencies of a number of nutrients. They included the minerals magnesium, zinc, and molybdenum; the amino acids tyrosine, proline and glycine (two amino acids needed for repair and rebuilding of damaged cartilage); and phenylalanine, methionine, and leucine (three amino acids required for the production of enkephalins, the brain's natural painkillers). So important is leucine in helping reduce pain that deficiencies of this amino acid are almost certain to cause hypersensitivity to pain. One patient who suffered from a serious leucine deficiency was actually given the nickname *Ouch!*, because he could barely stand to have anyone touch him without crying out in pain.

I increased Beth's dosages of the Quick-Start nutrient DL-phenylalanine to 2,500 mg, three times daily. I also directed her to take the following nutrients three times per day: tyrosine (1,500 mg), leucine (1,500 mg), and proline (1,000 mg). And I recommended that she use two heaping teaspoons of glycine powder each day. This substance can be used as a sweetener in beverages and on cereals and fruit, and the two teaspoons could be divided into smaller doses taken throughout the day. I directed her to supplement the Quick-Start mineral supplements she was already taking with 500 mg of magnesium glycinate, taken three times per day, and 30 mg of zinc methionate (in a product called Optizinc) in addition to the zinc in her Detoxification mineral supplements, taken twice daily.

Although I also treated Beth for two other conditions, I wanted to focus this account on her successful recovery from opioid use. Despite the fact that on two occasions she intentionally took more than her allowance of hydrocodone, her recovery progressed very smoothly. At the end of five weeks, she had stopped the use of opioids completely. After six weeks of treatment, she gradually tapered her use of Clonidine to the lowest available dosage. After eight weeks, she stopped using this medication completely.

Beth reported only minimal substance cravings, and the chronic joint pain with which she had lived for years diminished rapidly. After six weeks, she declared herself pain-free. Four weeks after that she said that she'd only thought she was pain-free, but that she must not have really known what pain-free meant, because she had even less pain now than she did then. As with most chronic pain patients who engage in a constructive program of joint healing, Beth realized that her pain was continuing to lessen all the time.

CONCLUSION

Beth's case brings up several important issues related to opioid use. First, it points out traditional medicine's tendency to mask unresolved conditions with painkillers rather than attempt to correct the problem causing the pain. The treatments she received, because they never gave her what she needed to heal the damaged cartilage that was causing her pain, actually led her into a reliance on highly addictive prescription painkilling drugs. Second, while Beth had tried acupuncture, massage, and chiropractic treatments, and while these treatments can be very successful, they almost never provide complete relief unless the true causes of the pain they would relieve are treated.

Like Beth, Tony might well have fallen "victim" to traditional approaches to medical problems. In his case, had he gone the traditional treatment route, he might well have been given a heroin substitute, such as methadone, which would have kept him "hooked." In fact, yet another "me too" drug, buprenorphine (marketed as Buprenex, Temgesic, Suboxone, and Subutex) has been approved for the "treatment" of heroin addiction. Not surprisingly, this drug's primary use, when it first came on the market, was as a painkiller. Now, however, opiate abusers can take it and tell the world that they're not on heroin any more. What they can't tell the world, however—although many drug companies and drug treatment facilities would like them to do so—is that they're no longer disrupting the production of endorphins and enkephalins their brains produce. Furthermore, the disruptions are virtually identical to those caused by the use of heroin.

It's very similar to the methadone phenomenon. When methadone was first introduced, it was hailed as the "magic bullet" for heroin addicts. It quickly became clear, however, that methadone, like heroin, was valued very highly by addicts as a substance of abuse. Methadone's effectiveness as a drug of abuse was confirmed by the fact that drug users would pay very well for it. Heroin users who attend methadone clinics seek ways to get additional doses of the substance, which they can then sell to others on the street. Despite the clear scientific evidence that methadone is nothing more than a legal form of heroin, and that its use in no way "cures" people of heroin addictions, methadone clinics flourish.

The Power Recovery Program provides a clear alternative to these approaches, because it not only treats the source of substance problems at the biochemical level, but it also seeks the true biochemical reasons why people seek to use substances in the first place. Only when these root causes are addressed can the need to use substances be eliminated.

14

Stopping the Use
of Marijuana

Marijuana achieves its effects because it contains cannabinoids, such as THC (which is short for *tetrahydrocannabinol*), which occupy receptors in the brain designed for the brain's cannabinoid neurotransmitters, such as anandamide. Anandamide might well be called "the brain's natural marijuana," and, as with all neurotransmitters, artificial stimulation of receptors causes a cutback in the brain's normal production of and responsiveness to this natural neurotransmitter. After using marijuana over a long period of time, habitual users can become dull, unmotivated, and memory-challenged in the absence of their drug of choice, probably because their brains are either no longer producing normal amounts of anandamide or they become less responsive to it. THC differs from many psychotropic substances in that it remains in the brains or users for a long time. In cases of chronic marijuana users, it often takes months before their normal, "pre-pot" selves re-emerge.

In fairness to its adherents, the life-damaging effects of marijuana addiction are unlike those of the drugs we have discussed so far. Marijuana use or abuse does not seem to increase the propensity for violence and criminality, nor does it exact the enormous toll in medical morbidity and mortality which is commonly caused by other substances. Marijuana is far more subtle in its life-damaging effects, and potentially far more devastating in a psychospiritual sense.

CULTURAL CAUSES OF MARIJUANA ABUSE

Among the lasting changes which emerged from the so-called "counter-culture" of the 1960s and 1970s was the semi-legitimization of recreation-al drug use, particularly of marijuana, mescaline, LSD, and other psychedelic substances. Those who touted these substances as "mind-expanding" cited their use by North and South American indigenous peo-ples to induce visions, particularly in their religious ceremonies. A new classification, psychedelic music, sprang up as part of the phenomenon which saw both musicians and audiences alike focus on the use of these drugs in both the creation and the appreciation of a certain kind of rock music. The posters advertising concerts by these bands are testimony to the changes in consciousness psychedelic drugs were purported to induce.

The word anandamide, which represents the brain's "natural cannabi-noid," is taken from the Sanskrit word *ananda,* which roughly translates to "bliss" or "delight." Thus marijuana has attracted spiritual seekers who also are often attracted to other paths to "truth" and self-discovery. The cannabinoids in marijuana work by inhibiting the release of most neuro-transmitters, which can have the effect of slowing down, indeed, nearly stopping, the normal "stream of consciousness" and taking its users on an express route directly to "the now" to get a fleeting glimpse of the inner peace which meditators can only achieve incrementally through hard work over years. However, seasoned psychotherapists, pastoral coun-selors, meditation teachers, and those who have seriously investigated spirituality nearly universally agree that the road to psychospiritual growth is long, difficult, and sometimes tedious, and that despite the mar-vels of cannabis, designer drugs, psychedelics, and psychopharmacology, it is ultimately achieved by taking full self-responsibility for one's thoughts, feelings, and behaviors and avoiding shortcuts such as the chronic use of drugs.

Although all the so-called "psychedelic" drugs I've mentioned are potentially addictive, by far the one whose short- and long-term abuse negatively affects the greatest number of people is marijuana. Its ready availability, coupled with the fact that it has gained a measure of social acceptance and has many defenders, make it the most likely substance of abuse among teenagers and young adults. But marijuana is not attractive only to "seekers" and the young. There are also significant numbers of adults between the ages of 35 and 60 who have long histories of marijuana abuse. It's these two groups of users I've chosen to focus on in the case histories that follow.

CASCADE EFFECT CONDITIONS RESULTING FROM LONG-TERM MARIJUANA ABUSE

Many of the long-term cascade effect symptoms of marijuana abuse—including loss of focus and motivation—are familiar to most people. Below is a discussion of a number of these symptoms:

Deficiencies of essential fatty acids, especially phospholipids derived from organ meats, legumes, and eggs, are both precursors to and results of heavy marijuana use. The junk food cravings commonly experienced by marijuana users often contribute to dietary imbalances, especially to deficiencies of essential fatty acids, animal fat, and phospholipids. Marijuana users may be especially vulnerable to this because THC, the psychotropic compound in marijuana, is fat soluble and can disrupt the normal repair and maintenance of cell membranes. In addition, the overconsumption of junk food which so often accompanies marijuana use means that marijuana smokers take in a great deal of trans fats, exactly the wrong kind of fats for supporting cell membrane function and repair.

In the absence of their drug of choice, marijuana users can become listless and unmotivated (this is commonly known as "amotivational syndrome"), classic symptoms of *depression.* The retrograde signaling effect essentially inhibits many other neurotransmitter functions and causes many marijuana abusers to have low energy and to exhibit symptoms of depression.

These conditions are discussed in more detail in the following case histories. I want to emphasize that these case histories are meant to provide you with a *model* for seeking treatment and correcting any cascade effect symptoms your marijuana abuse may have caused. These secondary conditions, many of which can become very serious if left uncorrected, develop as a result of many factors, including genetics, stress levels, diet, and exposure to toxins. The best way to determine the precise biochemical causes of cascade effect symptoms is to have biochemical testing done by a qualified lab.

LINDA L.: A PLACE IN THE CROWD

By the time the changes in the way she dressed and acted had begun to "sink in" for her parents, 16-year-old Linda L. was immersed in a culture of drug use and defiance. The changes had happened gradually over a period of about eighteen months. As Linda described it to me, she and her friends were "tentative" at first, somewhat afraid to "get into drugs." Their tentativeness didn't last very long, however. Within a few months, Linda and her friends were rapidly adapting to new experiences. "Not everybody came along for the ride," Linda told me. "Three of my best friends dropped me because I started using drugs. I figured, okay, so what? They don't know what they're missing, and it's not my job to tell them, right?"

What her friends missed amounted to nothing less than a complete personality "makeover." From a young lady who was friendly, despite being somewhat shy, and who made honor roll every marking period, Linda was transformed into a sullen, sloppy girl who expressed disdain for everything from "nice clothes" to schoolwork. She used the newfound freedom her recently acquired driver's license gave her to expand her territory. She often drove groups of her friends around to parties, and they began to connect with other kids who had similar outlooks and similar approaches to having a good time. She often snuck out late at night during the week to be with her friends, sometimes staying out until 4:00 am or 5:00 am, driving around and getting high. Beer and marijuana were their primary substances of abuse. She and her friends began to get high on marijuana every day before classes, and Linda confessed to me that she spent each day "pretty much spaced out."

Her father told me that when he'd found a marijuana pipe in the back seat of the car, Linda had said, "That's where that got to. Bobby's been looking for that for two days." He said that he knew "deep down" that the pipe was probably hers, but he just couldn't confront her. "I didn't want to have to find out that my daughter was using drugs, even though it was pretty obvious she was. I guess I didn't know how to deal with it."

Linda's parents had brought her to see me after a harrowing incident. One night when she was partying with friends, Linda smoked some marijuana that had been laced with PCP, or "angel dust." This substance triggered a psychotic episode in Linda. She became irrational and violent, running through the house where the party was being held screaming and striking out at other people. Someone at the party called 911, and police cars and an ambulance arrived within ten minutes. Linda was rushed to the emergency room of a nearby hospital, where the anti-psychotic drug Haldol was administered. During her three-day convalescence in the hospital, Linda's doctor added Paxil, "to treat her depression," as he put it, to the Haldol she was taking.

I sensed that her recent drug experience and hospitalization had gotten Linda's attention and that she was at least ready to listen to what I had to say. It's an unfortunate fact that, in too many cases, it takes an incident such as Linda's to get young people to wake up to the potential dangers of drug use. By the time she came to see me, Linda was already tapering her use of Haldol and Paxil. The biochemical imbalances that were at the root of her marijuana use would be our primary focus.

As it turned out, there was a single glaring deficiency that may have been the root cause of Linda's taking so readily to marijuana. That cause was a severe deficiency in both Omega 3 and Omega 6 fatty acids (EFAs), animal fats and butter (sources of arachidonic acid), and lecithin (a source of phospholipids) in her diet. American diets, especially those of young people who seem to take readily to the low-fat diet craze, are dangerously deficient in essential fatty acids, phospholipids, and/or EFAs. Young women are often especially vulnerable to low-fat propaganda, because they believe they must conform to the cultural standard of anorexic-looking bodies perpetuated by super-thin fashion models. These substances are derived from fish such as salmon and from uncooked nuts and seeds, as well as from lecithin-containing foods such as legumes (including tofu, peas, beans, and lentils), and from eggs and liver. I've found, through the results of testing a large group of patients, that essential fatty acid deficiencies are virtually always present in those who develop both acute and long-term marijuana problems. Perhaps because Linda's levels of other nutrients —including amino acids, minerals, and vitamins—for which we tested were within normal limits, this one deficiency stood out in sharp relief.

Her treatment included 2,000 mg of purified and concentrated Omega 3 fish oils, in the form of a product called OptiEPA, taken twice per day. Withdrawal from marijuana often mimics depression, because it leaves its users listless and dull, and the OptiEPA would help Linda cope with these symptoms. I also prescribed 2,000 mg of borage oil, taken twice daily. The

Omega 6 fatty acids in borage are a precursor in the production of the brain's natural anandamide and would help Linda restart that process. Finally, I directed Linda to take 3,000 mg of purified lecithin and 100 mg of phosphatidyl serine, a substance necessary for the maintenance and repair of brain cells, each twice per day. I recommended that she take a multi-mineral supplement and a B-vitamin supplement twice each day as well. Making sure she had the required amounts of vitamins and minerals would help her body do the cellular repair work that needed to be done.

I educated Linda and her parents about the dangers of empty calories and carbohydrates, and the fact that carbohydrates are the cause of fatty weight gain. I advised her to eat dense, high-protein, high-fat foods, and to consume lots of organic butter. The arachidonic acid in animal fats, combined with lecithin and lecithin-containing foods like eggs, liver, and beans, would provide the precursors for her to synthesize anandamide and other natural cannabinoids, something which she had been incapable of doing because of the absence of the nutrients in these foods.

The full regeneration of Linda's brain chemistry took the better part of six months. In no small part because of her harrowing experience, Linda lost the urge to "party." While she attended school regularly, she didn't participate in any after-school activities. She stayed around the house and, as she told it, "kind of took stock." Her memory and motivation returned to normal within about three months, she told me on a follow-up visit, but she didn't feel like seeing any friends, old or new. She finally came out of her shell, her father told me privately, when a boy who had just moved into their school district began to take an interest in her. When she discovered that he went to their church, and that he was a member of the church's youth fellowship, Linda decided that maybe she'd get back into that group. She also decided that she'd neglected her studies for too long, and that she'd be back on the honor roll soon, "just to make sure I haven't lost the touch."

I don't mean to make it appear as though a sudden interest in boys was what sparked Linda's recovery. In fact, the opposite is more likely true: The restoration of her natural ability to produce anandamide is likely what helped rekindle her interest in boys. She and her new boyfriend hung around together for a while, but nothing "serious" developed from it. "That's just as well. There's plenty of fish in the sea," Linda told me. "Lucky for me," she added with a wink.

GEORGE C.: DRIFTING AND DREAMING

As he explained it to me, George C. "just sort of woke up one day" and realized that he'd been working on his novel for nearly a decade and had amassed "hundreds of pages that weren't worth the paper they were printed on." He also realized that his book had become both an excuse for maintaining a lifestyle built around getting high on marijuana and a symbol of the failure of that lifestyle. At 36, George had, in his words, "finally just gotten too old to keep kidding myself about what I was really doing." It wasn't that he didn't still aspire to be a published writer. And it wasn't that he didn't derive great satisfaction from his writing. It was, he said, "that the course I was pursuing wasn't moving me toward the goals I'd set for myself nearly fifteen years ago." He continued, "I'd heard the phrase, 'Tune in, turn on, drop out,' but I never thought much about it. Just a catch phrase from the sixties. But in a very real sense, that's what I did. Not consciously, you understand. It's just kind of what happened. It's ultimately where this kind of continual pot high that I've maintained for the past fifteen years has taken me. It set me adrift. I need to get back on course."

One of George's biggest problems was admitting that he had a "problem" with marijuana. "It was always talked about as kind of a harmless drug. You know, you could get a nice buzz from it, and there weren't any, like, hangovers or anything like that. But I can tell you, it's not really harmless at all. It can put you in a place where the things that really should matter just don't. And that's dangerous. You know, deep down I do want to do something to make a positive difference in the way things are. But you have to care, you have to commit, in order to do that. And I've let a drug problem keep me from doing both of those things."

When his father passed away seven years ago, George moved back in with his mother, giving up the small apartment that had been, since he moved into it five years earlier, something of a symbol of the independence he was seeking. At the same time, since he no longer needed to pay rent, he cut down to a bare minimum the number of hours he worked at his part-time job. "Just enough to buy pot," he said ruefully. "That's all I needed."

George's diet, unlike those of many marijuana users, was adequate. His mother prepared most of his meals, and she was conscientious about the food they ate. George even referred to her as "something of a health nut." But George's case points up the fact that even in cases where dietary insufficiencies are not among the primary causes of biochemical imbalances, imbalances can still occur. It is extremely difficult to derive sufficient amounts of the nutrients needed to achieve and maintain biochemical health without using nutritional supplements, especially if you're a substance user.

Because George did not have health insurance, and because he couldn't afford to pay for diagnostic tests out of pocket, he went ahead without testing. Although in most cases of serious, long-term substance use I don't recommend proceeding without diagnostic tests, I felt that there were several factors that made it appropriate in George's case. First—and this *does* apply to all cases—the nutrients I would prescribe could have only positive effects, even if they didn't address all of George's nutritional deficiencies. Second, George, unlike many long-term substance users, was apparently in good health. Aside from a chronic cough that his smoking caused, he was symptom-free. Habitual marijuana use was far and away the main problem he needed to address, and the nutritional supplement protocol I prescribed for him was essentially identical to the one I had prescribed for Linda.

George didn't get rid of the marijuana remaining in his "stash," but he did resolve not to buy any more when he ran out. He told me rather sheepishly, "To be honest, I didn't know what I was going to do if I couldn't smoke, but I didn't want to break my promise to myself not to buy any more pot. So I cut down. I'm ashamed to admit this, but the reason I cut down was to make my supply last as long as possible."

What George didn't realize was that cutting down was, no pun intended, just what the doctor ordered. It takes time for brain tissue to rebuild itself and to restore its capability to produce anandamide and other natural cannabinoids, and until the rebuilding process is well under way, the need to smoke marijuana can remain fairly strong. Cutting down on the amount smoked gives neurons a better chance to get started with rebuilding. George's initial reduction was from smoking three to four "joints" per day to smoking one per day. As his supply dwindled, he found himself smoking three or four times per week, and, shortly after that, once or twice per week. Then the inevitable happened: He ran out. More significant, however, and definitely not inevitable, was the fact that he did keep his resolution. He didn't buy more pot. When he stopped using the substance altogether, he found that he had made his supply last for more than six weeks.

George noticed several things within a week of completely stopping his marijuana use. "I had been brain-fogged," he said. "All the time. I'd been smoking so long I'd completely lost any sense that maybe I wasn't thinking very well. I used to think smoking pot made everything more vivid, and maybe it did at one time. But now I look around me and I'm seeing things, well, clearly. Literally. Everything is somehow in sharper focus, and my memory is much better."

But while being able to think and see more clearly represented a dramatic change in George's life, the return of his ability to "feel," to react with emotional honesty, was even more important. He had had a four-year, on-again off-again relationship with a woman who was very fond of him but who found his constant marijuana use unacceptable. "That she was even still in my life at all was something of a miracle," George told me. He went on to explain what had happened. "I realized," he said, "that I'd never . . . well, maybe 'never' is too strong a word . . . that all my feelings centered on myself. It happened with Susan. We were sitting and talking, and I was telling her about the changes that I felt were starting to happen because I'd quit smoking pot, and, well, I started to cry. I had the strangest mix of feelings. I was tremendously happy that I was doing something to turn my life around, and at the same time I felt unbearably sad, because I realized how much I'd lost, how much I'd missed."

Susan didn't accept the marriage proposal George offered that evening. She told him that the emotions of the moment were running a little too high to make that important a decision on the spot. But the tone of her voice told George what he really needed to know. And subsequent events, including their marriage and George's becoming first a "stringer," and eventually a full-time newspaper journalist, would be enough, for the time being, to enable George to label his quitting marijuana a resounding success.

CONCLUSION

There are several important points I'd like to make about the use of marijuana. First, the fact that marijuana very rarely triggers violent behavior, and the medical morbidity and mortality statistics associated with its use are not high, does not mean that it is the harmless recreational drug its defenders would have us believe it is. Although, strictly speaking, marijuana does not have the addictive potential of substances such as cocaine, Ritalin, and heroin, its effects are somewhat more insidious and difficult to articulate, and it is entirely possible to get "hooked" on pot. Smoking marijuana does disrupt neurotransmitter function, and it does bring about changes that impair users' abilities to function effectively. It is a psychotropic substance, and it does cause perceptual and behavioral changes. For that reason, its use is not to be taken lightly.

My second point touches on the use of psychotropic substances by children and adolescents, a subject that is close to my heart. I want to be very clear on one thing: The use of marijuana by children and adolescents can have profound negative consequences for brain development and lead to long-term intellectual and emotional dysfunction. This is because the human brain takes fully twenty to twenty-five years to develop to maturity. During this time, the brain is highly vulnerable to the effects of any psychotropic drugs, including marijuana. The reason for this is that the growth and connectivities of dendrites, which form the root branching system of neurons, depends on unrestrained freedom to form neuronal communication networks. Because the use of marijuana inhibits this process, it literally stunts brain growth and development. This is not to say that the use of marijuana is not detrimental to adults as well, because adults, especially older adults, depend on neuroplasticity to keep their nervous systems young and agile. It is, however, meant to emphasize the critical importance of eliminating the use of marijuana among young people.

It is critical that we as parents and as members of society recognize this and do everything in our power to ensure that our children and adolescents do not need to use these substances. Among the most effective things we can do —and I can't overstate the importance of what I'm going to recommend here—is to provide them with the nutritional "tools" their bodies and brains need to develop fully. Where marijuana is concerned, providing these tools means, overwhelmingly, making sure they are supplied with the nutrients, especially essential fatty acids from fish and raw seeds and nuts, phosophlipids from organ meats, legumes, eggs, and butter (I want to re-emphasize that everyone should consume organic butter), which they need for healthy brain development. Excessive marijuana use is usually associated with severe deficiencies of these essential fats, and reintroducing these nutrients into young people's diets can at least help to provide the necessary biochemical foundation for a healthy, drug-free life.

Finally, a word of caution to those defenders of marijuana. I urge you to consider deeply the consequences of marijuana abuse from a psychosocial perspective. In my experience, marijuana slams the door on psychospiritual growth, and chronic users like George often stop growing and maturing. Seeing one's life as a meaningful experience, a learning process which ultimately allows us to experience peace and wisdom and which enhances our ability to love and be loved, is the true spiritual path, and traveling that path can only be done without the use of psychedelic substances like marijuana.

Part Four

America's "Other" Drug Problem and the Problem of Environmental Toxicity

In the 1960s and 1970s, when Medicare and Medicaid legislation was first being enacted, there were no provisions made to cover payment for prescription drugs. The reason for this was simple: The cost of prescription drugs was such a small percentage of overall medical costs that it was not deemed necessary. The drug industry was still the tail, the medical profession the dog.

Today, however, the roles are reversed. The drug industry is now the dog, and the medical profession its tail. So powerful has the drug industry become that *in most cases physicians no longer determine the treatments their patients will receive.* The drug industry does that for them. The drug industry not only tells physicians which drugs they should prescribe for specific sets of symptoms, but it also tells patients which drugs they should be taking, so that patients will tell their physicians which drugs to prescribe.

One of the consequences of the drug industry's taking over the practice of medicine is, of course, rising prescription drug costs. There's an old saying that explains the situation very well: "Never ask a barber if you need a haircut." The medical version of this is, "Never ask a drug company if you need a prescription." In both cases, you know the answer before you ask the question, and it's always *yes.* This bit of advice, however, points to an extremely serious situation: the corruption of medicine that exists today because of the ascendancy of the drug industry.

Indeed, prescription drugs may be the "cigarettes" of the late twentieth and early twenty-first centuries. The similarities are striking. The warning labels on most prescription drugs list debilitating, even life-threatening, side effects, much like the warning labels that have appeared on cigarette packs since the mid-1960s. And we're certainly entering the heyday of televised drug advertisements, much as the years from the late 1940s through the late 1970s were the heyday of print and televised cigarette ads. Cigarettes were even recommended by doctors during this time, and the American Medical Association supported the tobacco industry until well into the 1980s. We're even now beginning to see lawsuits against "big drugs" which detail the devastation that these toxic substances can create when they're indiscriminately prescribed. I find compelling evidence every day in the patients I treat to justify such a trend.

But, in addition to the capitulation of the medical profession to the drug industry, another problem, that of environmental toxins, has grown exponentially over the past half-century. Where, for instance, prior to World War II herbicides, pesticides, and artificial fertilizers were not used, after mid-century our food supply became increasingly compromised by these toxins. Moreover, the expulsion of toxins such as heavy metals into the environment has increased at an alarming rate, and the result has been that many people find themselves the victims of physical symptoms and behavioral problems caused by excess toxins they have ingested or absorbed, often unknowingly. Yet conventional medicine has not seemed even to acknowledge that such symptoms might have their origins in excess toxic load.

The following chapters differ somewhat from those in the previous section, because they deal not with problem behavior on the part of those who take drugs, but on the part of the physicians who prescribe them and the toxins that have crept into our lives unacknowledged. The concern in this section focuses on what we need to do to avoid falling into the prescription drug trap, as well as how to treat symptoms caused by our increasing exposure to toxins. Therefore, although I do discuss cascade effect symptoms, the real point of the following case histories is to enable you to understand the problems faced by people for whom the medical establishment has prescribed powerful and unnecessary addictive substances as treatment. Part Four's chapters will help you to avoid becoming a victim of conventional medicine's overwhelming propensity to "throw drugs at disorders," coupled with its inability to understand the physiological basis of so many medical symptoms.

You'll meet two patients of mine who were exposed to potentially addictive drugs by their physicians, and whose lives could well have been ruined, not to say ended, if they hadn't found their way to treatment which enabled them to overcome the misguided treatment of their primary physicians. You'll also meet three other patients whose lives had been disrupted by excess toxic load and who turned to self-medication to solve their problems.

I would like to offer a special note to parents. As you may have gathered, I find the indiscriminate, irresponsible, even negligent use of powerful, potentially addictive psychotropic drugs to treat children and adolescents for so-called "behavioral disorders" to be among the most disturbing developments in modern medicine. For that reason, I've devoted Chapter 16 to the dangers of using powerful psychotropic drugs such as Ritalin, Adderall, Prozac, and Paxil, among many others, to make children "behave." It's an issue that concerns all of us, especially parents seeking safe, effective treatments for children diagnosed with Attention Deficit Disorder (ADD) or Attention Deficit/Hyperactivity Disorder (ADHD). If you're the parent of a child who has been diagnosed as having one of these conditions or who has other behavioral or emotional problems, Chapter 16 is extremely important. I'll explain why your child is getting shortchanged by "shortcut medicine." More important, I'll show you how to get safe, effective treatment for behavioral disorders— treatment that avoids the use of these dangerous and addictive drugs by safely and naturally correcting the biochemical imbalances which are critical components in most childhood and adolescent behavioral disorders.

15

When Bad Prescription Drugs Happen to Good People

W hen I speak of the drug industry determining treatments for many disorders, as I did in the introduction to Part Four, I'm addressing the "what" of the problem and leaving the "how much" question unanswered. In fact, the enormity of the problem would have been unimaginable even fifteen or twenty years ago. It's very well illustrated in the following case history. As you'll see, Bonnie N. had abused alcohol for many years and had many of the cascade effect symptoms that alcoholic people have, and I deal with her treatment of those symptoms in her case history. But she had an even more immediate problem: the extraordinary number of prescription drugs her physician had prescribed. It's on this problem that I've focused most of my attention in this chapter.

BONNIE N.: THE POWER OF DETERMINATION . . . AND BIOCHEMICAL BALANCE

"These ain't workin'," Bonnie N. said with characteristic directness as she pushed two sheets of paper across my desk toward me. Bonnie came to my office "to give it another try," *it* being overcoming her drinking problem. At 51, Bonnie was bright, lively, and good-natured. "I *do* like a good time," she admitted during our first conversation. "It had just gotten to where I liked it too much and too often. I've got to slow down."

Her attempt to "slow down" involved checking into a drug and alcohol rehabilitation facility. She had completed her three-week "detoxification" stay at the hospital two weeks earlier. The "these" she referred to that weren't "working" were the prescription medications the attending physician at the clinic had prescribed when she left the hospital. He'd prescribed them in order to, in his words, keep Bonnie "on the right track." The papers in front of me contained a list of the drugs. As I looked them over, Bonnie asked, "I mean, is that right? Is that what I need to do to stay off alcohol? To be honest, it seems to me I'd be better off just stickin' with the alcohol. At least it makes you feel good for a while."

When she checked into the rehabilitation facility, Bonnie had listed numerous problems common to people who have been drinking excessively for years. Among her symptoms were upper and lower gastrointestinal problems, including a burning sensation just below her breastbone, bloating, gas, and alternating diarrhea and constipation. "Food and me don't get along so well anymore," she complained. "Either I can't keep it down or I can't get it to stay around long enough to do any good." She also complained of low energy levels, depression, migraine headaches, difficulty concentrating, poor memory, joint pain, sleep problems, and allergies, and she had high blood pressure. Bonnie estimated that she averaged six or eight drinks per day, less during the week, more on weekends. She hastened to add that she hadn't touched a drink in the two weeks since she'd left the rehabilitation hospital. She also added that it was a real struggle not to drink, simply because she felt "so lousy all the time." I asked how long she had been drinking. Bonnie dropped her gaze as she said, "Since I was legal." She let me do the calculation, which came out to be about thirty years.

While in many ways Bonnie is typical of people who habitually consume alcohol to excess, she's different in one important way: She's not what I call a "pious patient." By that I mean that she's not a patient who complies with her doctor's orders without questioning them if it seems as though they might lead to harmful consequences. One of her main complaints was that the medications she had been given not only didn't seem to be working, but they also were actually making her feel worse. And Bonnie told me that it felt like her doctors were trying to "break her spirit" when she tried to question them about her treatment. "They kept telling me it was my 'alcoholic resistance,' that's the phrase they used, that made me not want to take those drugs," she told me. While most patients quietly "take their medicine," placing complete faith in drugs and doctors to find the answer to their drinking problems, Bonnie's independent streak led her to question her treatment and to look for an alternative.

The drugs on her prescription medications list were intended to reduce or eliminate her symptoms. I want to share the list with you for several reasons. First, Bonnie's treatment is not atypical of the medical and addictions communities' approaches to the types of symptoms Bonnie exhibited. But an even more important reason, to my way of thinking, is to give you an idea of the difficulties faced by alcohol and drug abusers who honestly want to try to stop their substance use. In many cases, as Bonnie knew intuitively, the treatment is at least as bad as the "disease." Too often, as was certainly the case with Bonnie, it's worse.

Bonnie's physician had ordered her to take *thirteen* prescription medications to help her deal with her symptoms. I'll identify the drugs and give you a summary of the symptoms they're supposed to counteract, their possible side effects, and the biochemical disruptions they can cause.

Revia (Naltrexone) is a psychotropic substance that blocks endorphin/enkephalin receptors, thus altering the brain's normal response to alcohol. Let me explain how this happens. When you consume significant amounts of alcohol, a substance called acetaldehyde is produced as the alcohol is broken down. This substance reacts with other brain chemicals to produce another substance, called THIQ, which can occupy enkephalin/endorphin receptors to reduce pain and help make the alcohol "high" more pleasant. By interfering with the ability of THIQ to occupy these receptors, Revia significantly diminishes the "high" achieved by drinking. There's a nasty catch-22, however: *For Revia to work, the person taking it must drink alcohol!* The drug only works in the presence of alcohol, so some alcohol must be consumed before it takes effect. Side effects of Revia include gastrointestinal problems, liver toxicity, insomnia, anxiety, abdominal pain, nausea and vomiting, fatigue, joint and muscle pain, dizziness, skin rash, chills, and, in the words of one of my patients, "feeling dead."

Prevacid, prescribed for Bonnie's gastrointestinal problems, directly suppresses the secretion of gastric acid in the stomach. Since stomach acid triggers the release of other digestive enzymes, a reduction in stomach acid can effectively inactivate many of the digestive enzymes necessary to break down protein in the food we eat. This, in turn, leads to the underdigestion and malabsorption of proteins. In addition, a reduction in the production of stomach acid results in the malabsorption of minerals. Finally, stomach acid is one of the important barriers our bodies have against parasites and many harmful bacteria, which are killed in the stomach. Reducing the production of stomach acid can allow these organisms to pass into the intestinal tract, where their presence often triggers digestive problems. Side effects of Prevacid include diarrhea, indigestion, gas, rectal bleeding, vomiting, gastroenteritis, and ulcerative colitis.

Estrace (Estradiol) is a form of estrogen often prescribed as part of an estrogen replacement program for menopausal women. Its use is linked statistically to increases in breast and uterine cancers. Other potential risks of estradiol therapy include high blood pressure, gall bladder disease, blood clots, increased triglyceride levels, and fluid retention.

Claritin, an "allergy drug," is known as a tricyclic antihistamine. It achieves its effects by preventing white blood cells from releasing histamine, which, in addition to being a natural anti-allergenic substance produced by the body, also functions as a neurotransmitter. Potential side effects of taking Claritin include high blood pressure, migraine headaches, loss of appetite, vomiting, joint and muscle pain, anxiety, depression, insomnia, bronchitis, nosebleeds, sinusitis, loss of sexual desire, skin irritations, and urinary incontinence.

Prozac, which was prescribed for Bonnie's depression, is a serotonin-selective reuptake inhibitor. (Refer to Chapter 3 for a discussion of SSRIs.) In addition to disrupting the serotonin cycle, this drug can cause chills, high blood pressure, increased appetite leading to weight gain, nausea and vomiting, hemorrhages, agitation, confusion, amnesia, sleep disorders, ear pain and ringing in the ears, and the need to urinate frequently.

Propranolol (Inderol) was prescribed to reduce Bonnie's mild high blood pressure. Potential side effects of this drug include asthma, congestive heart failure, depression, insomnia, hallucinations, emotional instability, memory loss, nausea and vomiting, and diarrhea.

BuSpar was prescribed to alleviate Bonnie's anxiety. Possible side effects of taking BuSpar include dizziness, nausea, headache, lightheadedness, anxiety and depression (despite the fact that it is prescribed to alleviate these conditions), nightmares and hallucinations, seizures, ringing in the ears, sore throat, nasal congestion, and chest pain.

Benzonatate (Tessalon Perles) was prescribed to reduce Bonnie's "smoker's cough." Its potential side effects include asthma, closing up of the throat, cardiovascular collapse, headache, dizziness, constipation, gastrointestinal upset, and skin eruptions. Behavioral side effects of this drug include bizarre behavior, mental confusion, and hallucinations when prescribed in combination with other drugs.

Trazodone (Desyrel), which is another SSRI and thus further disrupts the serotonin cycle, usually causes sedation and was prescribed for Bonnie's insomnia. Its potential side effects include low blood pressure, severe allergic reactions, memory loss, chest pain, gas, hallucinations, blood in the urine, eczema, blurred vision, constipation, fatigue, headache, and anxiety.

Midrin is one of two painkillers prescribed for Bonnie's migraine headaches. It consists of acetaminophen (commercially best known as Tylenol) combined with Isometheptene Mucide, an amphetamine-like drug which directly occupies dopamine receptors, and Dichloralphenazone, which is a sedative. Isometheptene Mucide was apparently included to counteract the effects of Dichloralphenazone, or perhaps it was the other way around. Bonnie took no comfort from the knowledge that she could take this drug without having to worry about getting either too excited or too sleepy. Side effects can include worsening of glaucoma, high blood pressure, skin rashes, and worsening of cardiovascular disease.

Biaxin is a broad-spectrum antibiotic. Like most commonly prescribed antibiotics, Biaxin kills beneficial intestinal flora. In cases such as Bonnie's, when they're prescribed without provision for restoring the balance among intestinal bacteria, they often worsen gastrointestinal problems. Side effects of this drug can include severe colitis, diarrhea, nausea, headache, abdominal pain, hallucinations, insomnia, nightmares, ringing in the ears, heart arrhythmia, and psychotic episodes.

Cyproheptadine (Periactin), another drug prescribed for Bonnie's "allergic rhinitis" (runny nose), occupies both serotonin and histamine receptors. Its side effects can include sedation, dizziness, disturbed physical coordination, mental confusion, restlessness, anxiety, irritability, insomnia, convulsions, hallucinations, skin rashes, ringing in the ears, loss of appetite, nausea and vomiting, wheezing, fatigue, chills, and headache.

Finally, to help Bonnie get rid of her nicotine cravings and stop smoking, her physician prescribed . . . that's right: *nicotine.*

It may seem unbelievable that someone could be taking all thirteen of these prescription drugs, and it is hard for me to believe that this dangerous, potentially lethal combination of drugs was prescribed in good faith and with good intentions. But the fact is that this is not an isolated case. Combinations of drugs such as the ones prescribed for Bonnie are becoming the rule rather than the exception, not only in the treatment of patients with drug and/or alcohol problems, but for patients who have many of the same symptoms Bonnie had, even though they are not substance abusers. In other words, you don't have to be a recovering substance user to get caught in the prescription drug trap.

In fact, the problem of over-prescribing drugs to substance abusers has become so prevalent today that so-called detoxification facilities have actually become "retoxification" facilities. This is in no small part because drug companies have won the "ad wars" against their competitors, the manufacturers of cigarettes and alcohol. Pharmaceutical companies can advertise their products on television, the other two can't, and drug manufacturers are reaping a financial windfall from this competitive advantage over the other two legal providers of addictive substances.

As you can see, each of these drugs by itself has the potential to cause severe biochemical imbalances and put patients at serious risk for profound and dangerous side effects. When they're prescribed in combination with each other, as in Bonnie's case, their disruptions of normal biochemical processes can be deadly. Seven of the thirteen drugs prescribed for Bonnie are powerful psychotropic substances, interacting directly with brain cells to disrupt the normal production, release, and reuptake of several key neurotransmitters. In this case, they were exacerbating existing and already serious biochemical imbalances which had developed as a result of Bonnie's excessive alcohol and cigarette consumption. To make matters worse, these drugs in combination almost guaranteed that, in addition to her problem with alcohol, Bonnie would become cross-addicted to her prescription medication.

Several of the drugs prescribed for Bonnie have effects that counteract those of other drugs on her list. Others have effects counter to those desired in Bonnie's treatment. For example, although she was being treated for depression, her physician prescribed the drug Propranolol, which has been shown to *cause* symptoms of depression in otherwise healthy people who take it.

Several of the drugs, including Claritin and Isometheptene Mucide, work by directly occupying dopamine receptors. Bonnie's dopamine cycle was being disrupted by three different drugs, each of which causes prolonged and unnatural stimulation. In addition, Prozac, BuSpar, Cyproheptadine, and Trazodone all disrupt the serotonin cycle. The use of these drugs in combination actually resulted in a severe cutback in Bonnie's production of serotonin, exactly the opposite of what she needed to help her cope with her depression.

Don't get me wrong. As I've pointed out in Chapter 6, withdrawal from alcohol can be accompanied by serious, even life-threatening complications. The use of drugs for periods of a few days to a few weeks during the early stages of withdrawal under medical supervision is often appropriate to counteract acute, short-term problems when there are no safer alternatives. Bonnie's alcohol problem was serious enough that she may have required drugs to help her through the early stages of withdrawal. But Bonnie faced months, even years, of continuing to use drugs which would ostensibly aid her recovery, and because of them her mental and physical health, even her life, were at risk.

For instance, if Bonnie were to relapse and begin drinking heavily again (which she would need to do to enable Revia to work!), the alcohol in combination with the prescription drugs she was taking would put her at grave risk for acute respiratory arrest, to name just one of the several life-threatening consequences that she would face. A very high percentage of deaths from drug overdoses occur when alcohol is consumed in combination with other psychotropic drugs, either prescription or "recreational."

It was very important in Bonnie's case to reduce, and eventually eliminate, her intake of this potentially damaging combination of prescription drugs. At the same time, these substances are so powerful and so potentially addictive, and she was taking so many of them, I knew that we needed to proceed cautiously. I even considered having her readmitted to another drug and alcohol detoxification facility while she detoxified from the prescription drugs that she had been ordered to take at the original detoxification hospital! I chose to have her withdrawal supervised on an outpatient basis.

Bonnie's Quick-Start questionnaire results indicated that she was deficient in catecholamines, the "go-for-the-gusto" neurotransmitters which enable us to experience pleasure, to concentrate, and to be motivated. Several of the drugs she was taking disrupted her catecholamine cycle, and I prescribed the Quick-Start nutrients to correct her deficiency. In addition, I prescribed the Power Recovery Program Detoxification nutrients. Because of Bonnie's long-term excessive use of alcohol, I also knew that she would have several degenerative conditions which I would need to begin to address immediately with nutrients that went beyond the scope of the Power Recovery Program Quick-Start and Detoxification regimens. Let me review them briefly.

Magnesium glycinate: 1,500 mg with each meal and at bedtime. Every single person I've treated for long-term alcohol abuse has suffered from a deficiency of the mineral magnesium. Magnesium is one of the most important life supporting nutrients. As I've noted in other places, it is involved in more than 400 different biochemical reactions, and it functions as a relaxant for neurons and muscles. Magnesium deficiencies are common in people who suffer from insomnia, high blood pressure, and migraine headaches, all of which were among the conditions for which Bonnie was being treated. Magnesium glycinate, the particular form of magnesium which I prescribed for Bonnie, consists of a magnesium molecule in combination with two molecules of the amino acid glycine. I prescribed this nutrient in addition to that in her Quick-Start mineral supplement because magnesium is especially easily absorbed and utilized by the body in this form. In addition, glycine itself is an important relaxing neurotransmitter.

OptiEPA: 3,000 mg, twice per day. Deficiencies in Omega 3 essential fatty acids are among the causes of depression, migraine headaches, and high blood pressure, and I prescribed them to help treat these conditions in Bonnie. Like a high percentage of alcohol abusers, Bonnie was almost certain to have inadequate levels of these critical nutrients.

Quercetin: 1,000 mg, three times per day. The nutrient quercetin is a citrus bioflavenoid which, in combination with bromelain, a digestive enzyme extracted from pineapple, has extraordinary antihistamine qualities. Unlike prescription antihistamine drugs, which often have dangerous side effects, these nutrients are safe. They provide relief from allergic symptoms with none of the typical side effects, such as drowsiness, dry mouth, and lightheadedness, that are associated with the use of prescription antihistamines. These nutrients can be purchased separately or in combination.

Bromelain: 1,000 mg, three times per day. The nutrient bromelain is a digestive enzyme extracted from pineapple which, in combination with quercetin, a citrus bioflavenoid, has extraordinary antihistamine qualities. Unlike prescription antihistamine drugs, which often have dangerous side effects, these nutrients are safe. They provide relief from allergic symptoms with none of the typical side effects, such as drowsiness, dry mouth, and lightheadedness, that are associated with the use of prescription antihistamines. These nutrients can be purchased separately or in combination.

During the two weeks until her second appointment to review her test results, Bonnie began to taper her dosages of prescription drugs. I had recommended that she take four to six weeks to totally eliminate them, and that she try to reduce her dosages by one-third before our next appointment. I arranged for a trained nurse to see Bonnie at her house every other day to make sure she didn't have problems withdrawing.

Being the determined patient she was, Bonnie tapered her prescription drugs much faster than I normally recommend. By the time of her second appointment, which was actually three weeks later, she had stopped using her medication altogether, except for Propranolol, which I had indicated would be very dangerous to stop abruptly. "My daddy always told me I had a strong constitution," she said, "so I decided this was the right time to make use of it." Her symptoms had by no means gone away. She had had two migraine headaches and still had trouble getting to sleep at night. She was also, in her words, "tired all the time, but who isn't when they don't sleep right?"

Despite this, Bonnie was determined, as she put it, "to ride this thing into the ground." She elaborated on what she meant: "I finally decided I wasn't going to give in to the alcohol any more, and I'm damn sure not going to give in to those prescription drugs. I like the idea of doing it on my own. Let me say that another way. I like the idea of finally having what I need to do it on my own."

Bonnie's Quick-Start questionnaires and the fact that several of the drugs she was taking disrupted the serotonin cycle made it almost certain that she was serotonin-deficient, and she had been taking 5HTP to help boost her serotonin level as part of her Quick-Start regimen. The results of her Amino Acid Analysis confirmed that she was seriously deficient in tyrosine, the amino acid required for catecholamine production, and I recommended that she boost her intake of this nutrient to 2,500 mg, taken three times per day. Like many other people who abuse alcohol, she also had low levels of the amino acid leucine, which is required in enkephalin production. I prescribed 2,500 mg of this nutrient to be taken twice per day.

Bonnie's Elemental Analysis confirmed that she was very deficient in magnesium, which she was already taking, both in her Quick-Start mineral supplements and the additional magnesium glycinate I'd prescribed. She was also deficient in zinc; however, she would be getting enough zinc in her Quick-Start mineral supplements to increase her baseline levels of this nutrient.

Bonnie's Comprehensive Digestive Analysis test showed that she had a serious overgrowth of *candida albicans,* one of the strains of yeast that inhabit our intestinal tract. She also was mildly allergic to dairy products, potatoes, and eggplant. Bonnie was taking *lactobacillus acidophilus* and *bifidus,* the beneficial intestinal flora that compete with yeast, as part of her Detoxification nutrients, and we would monitor her yeast levels in subsequent tests to make sure they were reduced to normal levels. I instructed her to eliminate the foods to which she was allergic for at least the next three months, until her digestive system had a chance to rebalance and heal itself.

It was nearly eight weeks before Bonnie noticed significant improvements. "Then," she explained, "I just woke up one morning and I felt better. A lot better. And then I realized it hadn't happened overnight. I was getting better a little at a time, every day, but I just couldn't quite see it. The changes were real small, and finally they just kind of added up to where you couldn't miss them."

Bonnie's case history is significant for a number of reasons. Bonnie is a very determined person, and this helped her immeasurably to recover from a serious alcohol problem. It's impossible for me to overstate the importance of determination in overcoming substance problems such as Bonnie's. In fact, I credit Bonnie's determination with helping her survive a traditional rehabilitation program. I say "survive" because the daunting array of powerful, toxic, potentially addictive psychotropic drugs that was prescribed for her by the hospital physician was enough in itself to break the will of a less determined person. Bonnie not only overcame an alcohol problem, she overcame a prescription drug problem that could have had negative consequences that were worse than those caused by alcohol.

Bonnie's words, spoken four months after she began treatment with me, sum up what I described to her as a *return to normalcy:* "I'm not sure if you could say I'm back to normal, because I'm not sure I ever knew what 'normal' was. But I'll tell you what, whatever I'm back to, it's a hell of a lot better than what I was used to." Virtually all of Bonnie's symptoms had been eliminated. She hadn't had a migraine headache for more than six weeks, and she was free of gastrointestinal symptoms. She was getting "six or seven straight hours of sleep pretty much every night," as she put it, and that hadn't happened for her "in a long, long time."

She was breathing "much better," she said. "Every now and again I see someone with one of those portable oxygen machines, and I think, 'That could've been me,' and it gives me chills." One of the reasons for this was that cigarettes had begun tasting, as she put it with her inimitable flair, "like I imagine road kill would taste if you tried to smoke it." She had cut down, she said, to "somewhere around half a pack a day, but I'm too ornery to quit altogether. What would people think?" Bonnie had found out that she could "party on ginger ale" and that having a good time now meant "just enjoying myself. I still like to have a good time," she went on, "but what makes for a good time doesn't have anything to do with drinking."

CONCLUSION

While Bonnie's case may at first seem extreme, it differs from those of others of my patients only because of the unusually large number of prescription psychotropic drugs she was instructed to take. I routinely treat patients whose physicians have prescribed from three to seven such substances, when the consequences of taking even one or two of them were potentially health- or life-threatening.

One of the important things that I hope you'll take away from Bonnie's case history is that taking even one prescription psychotropic drug to treat symptoms such as substance abuse, allergies, migraine headaches, gastrointestinal problems, depression, and anxiety, among many others, is an action which can have extremely serious negative consequences. As

I've said in the introduction to this part of the book, these drugs should be used only as a *last resort*, although most physicians and addictions treatment professionals prescribe them without so much as testing for the underlying physical causes of the symptoms they mask.

And I'd like to make one final point, about the seemingly large number of nutritional supplements I prescribed for Bonnie. One of the complaints I've heard from a number of patients (and this is something you may have been thinking yourself) goes something like this: "Gee, Doc, that seems like an awful lot of pills." When you find yourself looking at the Power Recover Program in this way, just think back to what Bonnie went through. She often took more than fifty pills each day, but the pills she was taking were not making her better. The mind-numbing array of psychotropic drugs (double meaning intended) she had to keep track of each day was daunting. Furthermore, they definitely caused enough mental confusion that she was at risk of taking more than the recommended doses of any of the drugs, simply because they made it very difficult for her to keep track of what she did take. So if you find yourself grumbling about the number of nutritional supplements you're taking, just remember that the Power Recovery Program nutrients are your key to restoring your physical and mental well-being and not a ticket to a lifetime dependency on psychotropic drugs. You'll also probably find that, as your mind becomes clearer, you won't have any problem at all remembering which supplements to take. Take it from Bonnie.

16

Readin', Writin', and Ritalin

Getting Kids Off Prescription Drugs

Don't think I'm exaggerating when I refer to Ritalin as "dangerous." The International Narcotics Control Board (INCB) has issued the following statement: "The abuse of methylphenidate [Ritalin] can lead to tolerance and severe psychological dependence. Psychotic episodes [and]violent and bizarre behavior have been reported." The United States Drug Enforcement Agency's list of the potential adverse effects of Ritalin includes "psychosis, depression, dizziness, insomnia, nervousness, irritability, and Tourette's Syndrome or other nervous tics." This chapter contains a case history to underscore these points and to demonstrate that, not only in this case but also in the overwhelming majority of cases, psychotropic drugs are not necessary to treat ADD and ADHD.

CONVENTIONAL MEDICINE: LEGALIZING COCAINE FOR KIDS

Let me present a situation and then ask you a question which might at first seem outrageous but which I think you'll ultimately find to be very reasonable. To start, let's propose that you have a son between the ages of 6 and 16 whose grades have been slipping because he has difficulty concentrating on his schoolwork. In addition, he has trouble sitting still in class for more than five or ten minutes at a time. Now let's suppose that a drug dealer approaches you on the street and says, "I've got just the thing that will get rid of your son's problems: Cocaine!" Would you take this drug dealer's advice and give your son cocaine to help him concentrate better and fidget less? Of course you wouldn't.

But let's modify the scenario only slightly. Again, your son has difficulty concentrating on his schoolwork and can't sit still in class for more
than five or ten minutes at a time. This time, however, his teacher, the
school psychologist, and your family physician say, "We've got just the
thing that will get rid of your son's problems: Cocaine!" Would you say
yes in this case? The terrifying reality is that millions and millions of parents do say *yes* when offered this "solution."

Of course, the cocaine which the family physician prescribes goes by
the brand name Ritalin, and while a Ritalin molecule differs somewhat
from a cocaine molecule, it has exactly the same effect on the human brain
as cocaine. In Chapter 3, I explained how cocaine acts on dopamine reuptake receptors in the brain. Ritalin acts on these receptors in *exactly the
same way* cocaine does. In fact, among people who habitually use cocaine
and amphetamines to get high, Ritalin is known as "the cognac of speed."
And the "cognac of speed" is being taken regularly by almost 15 percent
of American schoolchildren between the ages of 6 and 17 to treat the conditions known as Attention Deficit Disorder (ADD) and Attention
Deficit/Hyperactivity Disorder (ADHD). Ninety percent of the schoolchildren taking Ritalin are male, which translates to this stunning statis-
tic: *More than 10 percent of American schoolboys are taking this legalized form
of cocaine every day, in most cases with the approval of their parents, teachers,
and healthcare providers!*

What makes this appalling situation even worse is that in the vast
majority of the diagnosed cases of ADD and ADHD, *symptoms can be successfully treated without medication.* In other words, we're putting a significant percentage of our children at risk for brain damage, substance
problems, and chronic neurological disorders because physicians and
school personnel will not address the root causes of these symptoms.
Instead, they choose to prescribe drugs which, while in most cases they
temporarily reduce or eliminate the symptoms, can actually make the
conditions causing them worse over time.

The situation is very similar to those out of which the need to use cigarettes, alcohol, and drugs arises. Biochemical imbalances alter brain
chemistry and lead to emotional and behavioral problems. In this case,
however, the source of the dangerous, potentially addictive psychotropic
drugs which temporarily alleviate the symptoms is not a drug dealer, it's
the American educational and medical establishments working in tandem.

JOHN W.: TAKING ADVANTAGE OF THE SYSTEM

John W. was 15 years old and would begin his sophomore year in high school a month and a half from the day his parents first brought him to see me. John had always been an above average student, but his grades began to slip and his classroom behavior became increasingly disruptive during eighth grade. By the end of eighth grade, John, his parents, and his teachers were all glad that school was over and that John would have a chance to, as his father put it, "regroup over the summer and come back ready for ninth grade."

Summer vacation turned out to be anything but an opportunity to regroup. John's behavior became increasingly unpredictable. His mother said, "It seems like he just became an angry kid. You couldn't say a word to him without getting a lot of attitude back. I was actually afraid he might become physically violent toward me, although he never did. We didn't know what to do." Only three weeks into his freshman year, John had been suspended for threatening a teacher. It was clear that his problems were getting worse and not better.

The appointment at which the family physician diagnosed John as having ADHD lasted approximately six minutes. The doctor reviewed the opinions of John's teacher and the school psychologist and concurred after asking John a few questions. He prescribed 5 mg of Ritalin, to be taken three times per day, for John's ADHD symptoms, and 20 mg of Paxil, taken once per day, for his aggressive behavior.

Although John at first resisted taking Ritalin and Paxil, he soon acquiesced and became very cooperative. His behavior in the classroom improved noticeably, and he no longer acted aggressively towards his teachers and fellow students. By the end of the second grading period, his marks were on the rise. When his ADHD symptoms began to return after about ten weeks, his doctor doubled John's Ritalin dosage from 5 to 10 mg, three times per day. By the end of the first semester, John's dosage was up to 20 mg, three times per day. His behavior and schoolwork remained acceptable. He continued his daily dosage of Paxil as well.

His teachers and the family doctor were gratified that, despite his initial reluctance, John had finally begun to see the benefits of taking medication. What they didn't realize, however, was that John was not actually *taking* his Ritalin. At least not much of it. John had discovered what thousands of teenagers across America have learned: A 5 mg tablet of Ritalin can be sold for $5.00. John had faked a return of his ADD symptoms on three occasions in order to have his dosage increased. He still took Paxil, but the 40 to 60 mg of Ritalin that he managed to slip into his pocket without the school nurse's knowing it netted him more than $1,000.00 a month when he sold them to other students at his school. You see, what I neglected to mention at the beginning of this case history was that John had been arrested for selling a controlled substance, and his appointment with me was part of his court-ordered rehabilitation.

At our second meeting, after he had begun to feel more comfortable, John loosened up. "It was easy," he explained when I asked him how he worked his scam. "The kids line up for the stuff outside the nurse's office. The line goes halfway down the hall. No way they watch what you do. You just pretend like you're popping it in your mouth, swallow some water, off you go." John also explained that the kids he sold Ritalin to usually ground it up into a powder and snorted it. "Just like cocaine," he said, not realizing how true his words were. When I asked him why he didn't take more of the Ritalin himself, John, like most kids for whom the drug is prescribed, simply said that he didn't like the way it made him feel.

John's parents were surprised to discover that I didn't immediately recommend drugs and counseling to help their son with his "psychological problem." I explained to them that imbalances in their son's body chemistry were almost certainly the causes of John's behavior problems, and that the first step in John's treatment would be to assess the state of his biochemical health by means of a series of tests. After I had explained my approach, John's mother made this extremely insightful comment: "What you're saying is that there are any number of possible causes for behavior like John's, and that the school and our doctor treated my son with Ritalin and Paxil without even knowing what was wrong with him."

Unfortunately, that's exactly what I was saying, and that's exactly what was done. John's treatment was the medical equivalent of asking a patient with a sore throat a few questions and then, without bothering to take a throat culture, prescribing aspirin and throat lozenges to alleviate the symptoms. Your patient could have strep throat and become gravely ill while you blithely continued to practice medicine irresponsibly. When physicians fail to do exhaustive biochemical testing to determine the possible underlying causes of the symptoms of ADD and ADHD, they're simply being negligent, as negligent as an MD who fails to order a throat culture for a potential strep infection. The problem is that this kind of irresponsible conduct has become the norm in treating behavioral disorders among young people.

Like my other patients, John filled out the Power Recovery Program Quick-Start questionnaires. This is because, like many other patients I treat, John was attempting to recover from a substance problem. The disturbing aspect of John's substance use was that *he had been ordered by his teachers and the family physician to become a substance user.* He had very little choice in the matter. It was very much as if he had been told, "Take this drug because we're ignorant of any other ways to bring your behavior back to acceptability, and we'd rather have you risk brain damage and future substance problems than really look into what's wrong with you."

Because Paxil had actually lessened John's aggression, my suspicion was that his tendency toward aggressive behavior resulted from a serotonin deficiency, and his questionnaire results confirmed this. The fact that he was also taking some Ritalin, a drug that, like cocaine, temporarily provided dopamine stimulation and enabled him to concentrate, indicated that he was also probably dopamine-deficient. His Quick-Start questionnaire answers also confirmed this. I prescribed the Quick-Start nutrients for both dopamine and serotonin deficiencies, and got John started on the Power Recovery Program Detoxification nutrients as well. I also ordered a series of tests to pinpoint these and other conditions that were the causes of John's behavior problems.

John, his mother, and I reviewed the test results several weeks later. His Amino Acid Analysis did, in fact, reveal that John was deficient in both tryptophan and tyrosine, as his Quick-Start questionnaires had indicated. John's tyrosine deficiency would have made it very difficult for his brain to produce enough of the neurotransmitter dopamine to keep him alert, motivated, and focused. In addition, because Ritalin occupies dopamine reuptake receptors and causes the brain to have to continually produce new supplies of dopamine, the net effect of his occasionally taking Ritalin would have been to further deplete John's supplies of tyrosine. Medicating a dopamine-deficient person with Ritalin only makes the true causes of unacceptable behavior worse.

His tryptophan levels were so low that, under the best of circumstances, John's brain would have been unable to produce adequate amounts of serotonin. This was complicated by the fact that John's Elemental Analysis test revealed high levels of copper. Let me explain copper's role in brain chemistry, because the balance that needs to be maintained is quite delicate. Copper is required for the production of *noradrenaline,* another neurotransmitter in the catecholamine family which helps us stay alert and focused. Noradrenaline is made from dopamine, and low levels of copper are sometimes found in dopamine-deficient people. But too much of a good thing can, in this case, turn into a bad thing, because excessive copper actually inhibits the production of serotonin. High copper levels are very often at the root of aggressive and violent behavior, and, in John's case, they were certainly among the primary causes of his symptoms.

The Elemental Analysis also revealed that John had excessive levels of lead. "You mean he's got lead poisoning?" his mother exclaimed. "Why didn't they find that?" I explained that lead toxicity usually does not show up in blood tests, because lead doesn't stay in the bloodstream for long periods of time. Instead it tends to bind to bodily tissues, especially hair. Because of this, the presence of high lead levels in chronic cases, such as John's, can only be determined by testing hair samples. I know of very few doctors who are aware of this, and, in fact, New York State has recently banned the use of hair testing as a method for determining levels of toxic minerals. New York is the only state in the United States to ban this type of testing, and by doing so the state almost guarantees that tens of thousands of cases of chronic heavy metal toxicity in children will go undetected and uncorrected. High levels of lead, by the way, are among the primary contributors to ADD and ADHD symptoms.

John's Fatty Acid Analysis test revealed serious deficiencies in Omega 3 fatty acids. I explained to John and his mother that deficiencies in these nutrients can cause cell membranes in the brain (and in other parts of the body) to lose flexibility, and that loss of flexibility impairs brain function. I prescribed 3,000 mg of OptiEPA, which is rich in Omega 3 fatty acids, to be taken three times per day.

John's recovery was rapid. Like many young people, he was very resilient once his body and brain had the nutrients they needed to detoxify and rebalance themselves. As a result of replenishing critical nutrients that were in short supply, John began to perform at very high levels in the classroom. In addition, he was able to achieve a stunning two-standard deviation improvement in his results on Intermediate Visual and Auditory, Continuous Performance testing, tests which measure physiological capabilities in children and adolescents. With normal copper levels restored, he gradually tapered and finally eliminated his Paxil use without experiencing a return of his aggressive tendencies.

John summed it up precisely when he said, "Every once in a while I walk past that line of people outside the nurse's office, and I think, 'Man, that used to be me!' And I can tell you that I'm seriously glad it isn't me anymore." His sense of humor had returned along with his zest for life since he'd stopped taking Ritalin and Paxil, and it surfaced in his parting comment, delivered with a wry and knowing smile: "I do miss the money, though." He paused for a beat before adding, "Just kidding!"

John's case history is true. That in itself would be bad enough, but it doesn't stop there. It's not only true, but it's also quite typical. I have personally treated other patients who not only took Ritalin but also "engineered" dosage increases so that they could sell what they didn't use to others, who used the drug to get high. And I've heard the story repeated by many middle and high school principals who deplore the abuse of Ritalin but who are relatively powerless to stop it in the face of overwhelming pressure from teachers, parents, psychologists, physicians, and, ultimately, drug companies.

AVOIDING THE RITALIN/ADDERALL/PAXIL NIGHTMARE FOR YOUR CHILDREN

The drug Ritalin (methylphenidate) was first approved for sale by the FDA in 1955. By the mid-1960s, its use for behavior control was spreading. By 1987, both Attention Deficit Disorder and Attention Deficit/Hyperactivity Disorder were approved by members of the American Psychiatric Association (APA) as "mental disorders," and entries describing them appear in the organization's *Diagnostic and Statistical Manual of Mental Disorders* *(DSM-IV)*. ADHD is deemed to be present when a child meets a specified number of the behavioral criteria which are listed in the *DSM-IV*.

But while Ritalin continues to soar in popularity as the treatment of choice for ADD and ADHD in the United States (which, incidentally, buys and uses 90 percent of the Ritalin sold in the world), the World Health Organization (WHO) has been raising warning flags for years. As early as

1971, the WHO had categorized Ritalin as a Schedule II drug. This means that it is classed—along with morphine, opium, cocaine, and the heroin substitute methadone—as one of the *most addictive substances in medical usage.* The United States Department of Justice concurred, including Ritalin as a Schedule II drug in the Controlled Substances Act, while warning that it has a very high potential for abuse. Ritalin differs from many prescription psychotropic drugs in that it has not been superseded by later generations of drugs that perform its function better than it does. Like its illegal counterpart, cocaine, Ritalin never seems to go out of favor.

Any discussion of the use of Ritalin and other psychotropic drugs to treat ADD and ADHD symptoms in children must concern itself not only with the social and moral issues associated with the practice, but the biochemical consequences for young people of using this kind of drug. Let me first try to clearly state a few of the social and moral components of the issue.

First, if more than 10 percent of children between the ages of 6 and 17 in the United States are so ill that they need a drug as powerful as Ritalin, shouldn't we be more concerned than we are to get to the source of the problem rather than just treating its symptoms? The extremely large number of young people diagnosed with this "disorder" suggests that there is virtually a society-wide set of conditions that are causing such a high percentage of schoolchildren to need this drug.

Second, we must also ask, "Since when did the reduction of the symptoms of a condition such as ADD through the use of a powerful, potentially addictive psychotropic substance—a substance which is illegal on the street—become a desired outcome of medical intervention?" In the cases of ADD and ADHD especially, to take such an approach is no less than an admission of failure.

Over time, the use of Ritalin can cause chronic disturbances of neurotransmitter function, making the user dependent on the outside drug in order to maintain even a semblance of normal brain function. In other words, when Ritalin is prescribed for an extended period of time, a biochemical dependence most certainly can develop in those who use it. Put another way, Ritalin is a powerful mind-altering drug, and the children for whom it is prescribed can abuse it, just as they could abuse cocaine.

In the case history recounted here, I've given you just one example of the numerous potential causes of the behavioral symptoms that are so cavalierly labeled ADD and ADHD and treated with psychotropic drugs. It would be impossible to list even a small percentage of the potential bio-chemical causes for these symptoms, and I'll not try to do that here. I will strongly recommend this, however: As John's case history shows, there are now extremely accurate and sophisticated tests available to determine potential biochemical causes of ADD and ADHD symptoms. We also know how to correct those causes without resorting to psychotropic drugs, and numerous scientifically valid studies have demonstrated that correcting the underlying biochemical imbalances eliminates the behav-ioral problems associated with ADD and ADHD.

If your child has been diagnosed as having ADD or ADHD, and if pressure is being put on you to have him take Ritalin, I urge you and your pediatrician or family physician to make use of the many tests that are available. Based on the results of these tests, strategies for eliminating ADD and ADHD symptoms can be developed which restore the body's natural brain chemistry without relying on the use of powerful psy-chotropic drugs.

Family counseling may also be necessary to deal with serious psycho-logical problems that can accompany the behavioral symptoms, but in many cases I have found that when the underlying biochemical problems are corrected and the problem behavior is eliminated, many of what were wrongly assumed to be psychological problems also disappeared, or were at least reduced to the level of minor irritants which could be dealt with effectively either within the family or in the context of family therapy as they occurred.

But let me make one thing clear: I'm not saying teachers and admin-istrators should have to put up with disruptive behavior in class. Far from it! I am saying that the standard method of eliminating disruptive behav-ior through the use of powerful, potentially addictive psychotropic drugs must be stopped, and then be replaced by treatments that provide our children's bodies with the means to heal themselves.

I've taken educators and physicians to task, but teachers, school administrators, counselors, and physicians aren't the only guilty ones in this situation. Parents must often share the blame. In the many hun-dreds of successful cases I've been involved with, I've occasionally seen children's ADD and ADHD symptoms successfully eliminated using completely natural means to restore their biochemical balance, only to have the *parents* request that their children be put back on Ritalin. Their reasons in all cases have to do with the parents' images of what their children should be. The parents of two of the children said that, while their sons were getting very good grades as a result of all-natural treatments, they felt they would do even better academically with Ritalin. A third set of parents "liked" their son better when he was being treated with Ritalin rather than with natural substances, because he was "very polite and nice." I'm frankly at a loss to comment on this kind of parental behavior.

The doses of Ritalin given to most children, at least before they begin to develop a tolerance for the drug and need greater amounts to achieve the same abatement of symptoms, are technically not sufficient to cause significant physical dependence. What does happen, however, is that children taking these doses of Ritalin "withdraw" every night after the drugs they have taken during the day wear off. Each day, many families see a return of irritability, restlessness, and the inability to concentrate as the evening wears on and their children's brains are deprived of their "chemical crutch." Once this is pointed out to most parents, they realize that Ritalin is not "curing" their children of a "disease"; it is simply temporarily masking symptoms which return as soon as the effects of the drug wear off.

The understanding that ADD and ADHD are *not* diseases is critically important. A friend of mine once defined "disease" as "an excuse for drug companies to develop and market new toxic substances." I'm afraid that, in the case of ADD and ADHD, he's right on the money. ADD and ADHD are not diseases at all; they are merely convenient labels under which to group symptoms which, in most cases, respond to treatment with powerful stimulants. But I can tell you categorically that I have yet to treat a single person for ADD and/or ADHD whose symptoms were not ultimately caused by stress, malnutrition, digestive disorders, high toxic load, allergies, parasites, or some combination of these factors. In every case, once the true underlying biochemical causes of the symptoms were identified and treated, the symptoms went away. *I have not treated a single case of ADD or ADHD in which the prescription of powerful psychotropic drugs was necessary for the elimination of symptoms!*

CONCLUSION

In this chapter, I've concentrated on the drugs prescribed to counteract symptoms of ADD and ADHD in our children, because they represent the most immediate danger to the present and long-term mental and emotional stability of our young people. But the problem doesn't end with Ritalin and Adderall. Hundreds of thousands of children, in some cases as young as three years old, are taking antidepressant drugs such as Prozac and Paxil to reduce the symptoms of everything from "depression" to "antisocial behavior." In too many cases, the results are disastrous.

Not one of the ADD/ADHD kids I've treated wanted to be on drugs such as Ritalin; more importantly, they do not need to be. There are natural alternatives, based on the recent extraordinary advances in our knowledge of how the human body works at the biochemical level, which offer new hope to ADD and ADHD children, their parents and teachers, and to society in general.

17

High Toxic Load

Dealing With a Common Condition Associated With Substance Abuse

In a recent study which I conducted involving 105 inpatients being treated for substance use disorders, I found an astonishing level of heavy metal toxicity, including, especially, antimony, cadmium, and lead poisoning. The average levels of poisoning of these three metals in the patients who participated were far greater than the 95 percent (two standard deviations) level which is used as a "cutoff" level for defining a serious toxicity. This study strongly suggests that most individuals suffering from substance use disorders are seriously poisoned with heavy metals. Since heavy metal toxicity of this high degree usually takes many years to build up in the tissues, the study also suggests that a significant percentage of addicted people were likely poisoned before they ever started using drugs and alcohol. Perhaps toxic metal poisoning is causing psychiatric symptoms which an addicted person then tries to medicate away with alcohol and drugs.

For instance, studies have linked cadmium toxicity to alcoholism, schizophrenia, ADHD, learning disabilities, and low blood sugars (hypoglycemia). Lead toxicity is associated with adrenal insufficiency, allergies, anorexia, anxiety, arthritis (rheumatoid and osteoarthritis), attention deficit disorder, autism, back pain, behavioral disorders, depression, dyslexia, emotional instability, fatigue, hallucinations, headaches, hostility, hyperactivity, hypothyroidism, impotence, decreased IQ, insomnia, irritability, joint pain, learning disability, liver dysfunction, loss of will, memory loss (long-term), menstrual problems, mood swings, multiple sclerosis, nightmares, psychosis, restlessness, retardation, schizophrenia, and seizures.

Less is known about antimony, but all three of these metals—cadmium, lead, and antimony—cause a wide array of medical problems.

The following case histories will help you understand more about the primary causes and some of the effects of high toxic load and about how the Power Recovery Program Detoxification nutrients work at the cellular and molecular levels to enhance your ability to get rid of accumulated toxins. Keep in mind that excess toxicity can manifest itself in many ways and that these case histories are just three examples of the kinds of conditions that can result.

MARIE M.: DEALING WITH FATIGUE AND MOOD DISORDERS

"I feel like life is cheating me," Marie complained during our first appointment. "I'm only 48 years old, but it seems like I'm always tired," she went on. "And if I'm not tired, I've got a headache. And if it's not one or the other, it's both. I don't know what I'm going to do. I just kind of feel *anxious* all the time." Marie also reported that she frequently experienced numbness and tingling in her arms and legs, and that she sometimes had problems with "brain fog." Marie had a history of moderately heavy alcohol use (she averaged "about four drinks a day"), and she had occasionally smoked marijuana and used cocaine at parties. When I first met with her, however, she had not used alcohol or drugs for more than a year. "It got to the point where all it did was make me feel worse," she said, "and feeling worse is not something I need in my life."

Marie's family physician had ordered blood chemistry diagnostic tests and thyroid function tests. When the results of these tests revealed no abnormalities, the doctor suggested she try psychotherapy. After three months of therapy, her therapist recommended Prozac, for which her doctor gave her a prescription. She took the drug for several months, with no noticeable changes in how she felt. Because of her history of alcohol use, she had begun to wonder if she was an alcoholic. "I've heard you never get over alcoholism, and I thought maybe that was my problem." I explained to her that, although she had perhaps abused alcohol, the fact that she could voluntarily quit suggested that she was not an alcoholic person. I also explained that if her symptoms had been caused only by the toxicity of alcohol and drugs, she would have begun feeling better within a few months of quitting.

The medical history questions she answered during her first appointment indicated that the primary neurotransmitter deficiency associated with Marie's alcohol use (and the mild depression she experienced) was of serotonin, and I prescribed the Quick-Start nutrients designed to help jump-start her serotonin production. At the same time, I shared with her my suspicion that, while she was almost certainly serotonin-deficient, there were also other factors contributing to her condition. Based on my experience in treating patients with Marie's symptoms, I suspected that the diagnostic tests I ordered would also reveal that Marie had a high toxic load. Since it would be ten days to two weeks before I'd see her again, I recommended that she begin taking the Power Recovery Program Detoxification nutrients as well.

When she returned to my office for her second appointment, Marie was somewhat discouraged. "I'm not sure if I'm following your program correctly," she said. "I'm afraid I really don't notice too much difference." When we reviewed the symptoms she had described to me during our first appointment, however, Marie changed her mind. She realized that she hadn't experienced numbness and tingling in her arms and legs for nearly a week. "It just went away, and I didn't even know it," she said, shaking her head and smiling tentatively.

She was still shaking her head as we began to review the results of her diagnostic tests. Two of them proved to be very revealing. First, tests to determine the levels of toxic elements in both hair and blood samples indicated dangerously high levels of mercury. Second, a test of amino acid levels in Marie's blood indicated that her levels of tryptophan, methionine, cysteine, and taurine were well below normal. It appeared very likely that mercury toxicity was the primary cause of Marie's symptoms.

"But I thought my doctor did a whole battery of blood tests," Marie said. "Why didn't he find out that I had high levels of mercury? I mean, that's pretty serious, right?" I told her that it was indeed "pretty serious." As I explained to her that most physicians do not routinely test for heavy metal toxicity, even when presented with symptoms such as hers which are often caused by heavy metal poisoning, she began to shake her head again, this time in anger and disbelief.

I also explained that the amino acids methionine, cysteine, and taurine all contain the element sulfur, and that mercury combines readily with sulfur. Her low levels of sulfur-containing amino acids suggested that Marie's body was depleting its reserves of these nutrients as it tried to eliminate the excess mercury by means of a natural process called chelation. Our bodies use sulfur to combine with numerous toxic substances, including mercury, in order to prepare them for elimination. Chelation is one of the natural processes our bodies employ as part of detoxification. In this instance, once it has been chelated in the body, mercury can be more readily excreted. In cases of serious heavy metal toxicity such as Marie's, however, the ability to chelate toxic substances can be overwhelmed, and the substance can remain in our bodies in excessive quantities.

Because it interacts readily with sulfur, mercury often combines with proteins and enzymes which have sulfur-containing amino acids as part of their chemical structures. In doing so, it disables these proteins and enzymes and disrupts the biochemical processes of which they are necessary components. Headaches, memory loss, and chronic tiredness are very common symptoms in people with high levels of mercury or other heavy metals.

A significant percentage of patients I treat for substance abuse problems have symptoms caused in some part by heavy metal toxicity, with more than 50 percent of them showing high levels of mercury. For that reason, one of the most important functions of the Power Recovery Program Detoxification nutrients is assisting in the removal of heavy metals. One of the ways this is accomplished is through the replacement of sulfur nutrients, which are depleted not only in dealing with heavy metals but also with other toxins. Three specific Power Recovery Program Detoxification nutrients - alpha lipoic acid, methylsulfonylmethane (MSM), and glutathione - are specifically targeted to contribute sulfur to the detoxification process. I told Marie that, since tests had confirmed that mercury toxicity was a problem, she could safely double her daily dosage of these three nutrients to help hasten her detoxification.

There are several probable sources for mercury toxicity, including mercury amalgam dental fillings, tuna and swordfish, and (although this is not common) drinking water. Because of this, I recommended that Marie have a dental checkup, which she did. Her dentist found three older mercury amalgam fillings which had cracked and were almost certainly the source of the mercury in Marie's body. She chose to have them replaced with non-mercury fillings. In addition, I recommended that she add high-sulfur foods, including cilantro, garlic, broccoli, and parsley, to her diet, and that she avoid eating tuna and swordfish. Finally, I suggested that she install a water filter to remove any other potential heavy metal contaminants from her drinking water.

When Marie returned to my office four months later, she was, in her words, a "new person. I guess it wasn't life that was cheating me after all," she said. "I just had to find out what life needed from me to make living fun again. It turned out to be nutrients. Go figure." The results of her followup tests indicated her mercury levels were at acceptable levels, and, as a result, Marie's symptoms had all but completely disappeared. She had no desire for alcohol or other psychotropic substances. In fact, as she stated it, "I don't have any desire for any substance except those that make me feel good. Meaning nutrients. It's like I've been let out of prison."

RALPH C.: REPAIRING BARRIERS

Although Marie's case provides an example of someone who had a high toxic load despite the fact that her toxin "barriers" remained intact, many of my patients' problems result from breaks in their toxin barriers. The barriers which are critical in preventing toxins from entering our blood and lymph systems include the following:

• Stomach acid, which kills many potentially harmful bacteria and parasites in the food and water we consume.

• Digestive enzymes in the stomach and small intestines, which break down food into nutrient molecules that can be used by our cells.

• Beneficial intestinal flora, which compete with harmful bacteria, yeast, and parasites to maintain a healthy intestinal balance.

• The intestinal wall, which normally screens out toxins while allowing nutrient molecules to pass through to the blood and lymph.

• The immune system, which responds to foreign substances, including toxins and microorganisms which manage to pass through the first four barriers.

• The liver, which filters and removes toxins from nutrient-rich blood after it leaves the intestines.

When these barriers are intact, our natural ability to process and eliminate toxic substances usually enables us to live healthy lives. When any of them are compromised, serious problems can result, as the following case history demonstrates.

At 32, Ralph C. was a successful technical sales representative for a major company. He's bright, very personable, and, as he puts it, "a little like a pit bull when it comes to perseverance." He credits his success as a salesman in a competitive field to aggressiveness and determination. He also recognizes that these same traits may have played a part in his excessive substance use and, because of this, they might eventually have helped ruin his career.

Ralph's problem boiled down to the fact that he just didn't feel right. "And not just some of the time," he was quick to add. "I'm talking about most of the time. I have a good day maybe once a week. Maybe." When he first came to my office, Ralph had already been receiving medical treatment for gastrointestinal problems for more than four years. He suffered from bloating, alternating diarrhea and constipation, gas, and chronic intermittent abdominal pain which, he explained, his doctors had told him was "hard to pin down." He also complained of fatigue and mild depression, and he experienced sleep problems. "The most humiliating thing, though," he confessed, "was when I had to move my desk closer to the restroom. My problem got so bad sometimes that I was worried I just wouldn't make it to the bathroom on time."

Two gastroenterologists and three primary care doctors had evaluated Ralph, and he had undergone two full gastrointestinal workups, both of which included colonoscopies. The consensus was that Ralph was suffering from Irritable Bowel Syndrome (IBS). His doctors also agreed that they could do very little for him other than prescribe medication—which included the anti-inflammatory drugs Prednisone and Azulfidine—to relieve his symptoms. Ralph was also given a prescription for the SSRI Paxil (generic name *paroxetine*), which he did not take regularly, to relieve his symptoms of depression. Despite his health problems, Ralph rarely missed a day of work.

I noticed that his previous diagnostic tests indicated possible liver function problems, and I asked him about his alcohol use. He consumed an average of "five or six drinks a day," he said. He had suspected that alcohol could be a factor in his intestinal problems, and he had quit drinking for three months to see if he could get relief. However, even when he was not drinking, he continued to have bouts of Irritable Bowel Syndrome, though they were not quite as severe as when he was drinking.

The diagnostic tests I ordered for Ralph indicated that his intestinal problems resulted from serious breakdowns in his body's barriers against toxins. His pancreas was producing insufficient amounts of the digestive enzyme chymotrypsin, and his levels of *lactobacillus acidophilus* and *bifidus*, two beneficial intestinal flora, were very low. This had resulted in a yeast overgrowth that contributed to his problems.

The tests also revealed that Ralph had several food allergies, which were likely caused by Leaky Gut Syndrome, a condition not uncommon in alcoholic people. The term *leaky gut* refers to a condition in which the powerful bonds that hold the cells lining the intestinal walls together weaken, allowing partially digested food molecules and toxins created by harmful intestinal flora to "leak" through into the bloodstream without passing through the cells themselves. The body's immune system perceives these substances as antigens and an immune system response is initiated. This response is the same as that mounted against any foreign substance that enters the circulation. The Allergy Profile test I ordered for Ralph indicated that his immune system was producing antibodies against wheat, milk, peanuts, and eggs. These foods were entering his bloodstream before they had been completely broken down into molecules which his body could absorb normally, and were therefore causing an immune system response. This, in turn, had contributed to a condition of chronic immune stress, which had made Ralph's symptoms worse.

Since the medical history form he filled out at his first visit indicated deficiencies of both dopamine and endorphins, Ralph had been taking the Quick-Start nutrients to correct those conditions. I had also prescribed the Power Recovery Program Detoxification nutrients. As his test results made clear, Ralph's detoxification needs focused on healing his intestinal tract. One of the Power Recovery Program Detoxification nutrients, phosphatidyl choline, would be important in helping strengthen the cell membranes of his intestinal walls. Two others, *bifidus* and *lactobacillus acidophilus*, would help restore his beneficial intestinal flora to normal levels and would help combat his yeast overgrowth. In addition, sulfur nutrients would help support the processing of toxins in the liver, just as they had for Marie. This would support Ralph's ability to remove toxins as the integrity of his intestinal walls was restored and his digestive function returned to normal.

It's important to note that while both Ralph and Marie needed sulfur nutrients to improve their liver function, the source of their toxins was very different. Marie's high toxic load was from an external source, the mercury from old dental fillings, while Ralph's toxins, undigested nutrient molecules and toxic byproducts of yeast metabolism, were from an internal source. It's partly because toxic load can come from so many sources, both external and internal, that I recommend the Power Recovery Program Detoxification nutrients to virtually all my patients.

I did not prescribe an antifungal drug which would target Ralph's yeast overgrowth. Instead, I recommended that Ralph avoid eating any of the foods to which he had developed allergies, and that he follow a high-protein, low-carbohydrate diet to help eliminate the sugars on which yeast feed. Reducing sugar intake (and thus starving the yeast) and reestablishing *lactobacillus acidophilus* and *bifidus,* two beneficial intestinal flora which compete with yeast and help prevent yeast overgrowth, would be our initial strategy. If this did not eliminate Ralph's yeast problem, I suggested we could consider using antibiotics. Unlike many physicians, I consider the use of antibiotics and antifungals a last resort. Except in cases of acute infections which must be treated immediately, I find that providing patients with what their bodies need to strengthen their ability to combat these conditions naturally is not only safer, but it is also much more successful over the long term. Finally, I also strongly recommended that Ralph not use alcohol for the next three to six months as his body healed itself.

Ralph did better than that. In the two years since he completed the nutritional treatments I prescribed, he's had "maybe ten or twelve drinks." He goes on to explain, "Once in a great while I have a glass of wine with dinner, and I've been at two wedding receptions where they gave champagne toasts. It was a real good feeling, to be able to toast the bride and groom and know that taking one drink didn't mean I'd feel like I had to keep going back to the bar all afternoon. The thing is, it's not a problem now. I can take it or leave it. I was always afraid to quit drinking, because I thought I'd be in this constant struggle not to relapse. It's not an issue. I can enjoy a drink with friends and not worry. I don't need to cover up feeling bad with booze."

MARGARET R.: RESTORING IMPAIRED LIVER FUNCTION

Margaret R.'s problem did not center on alcohol or other so-called "recreational" drugs. At 29, although she had used alcohol moderately, her real problems, she told me, were depression and anxiety. She explained that her symptoms had gradually worsened over the past four or five years, to the point where she and her boyfriend, Jeff, had broken off their engagement. "I just could barely function in the relationship," she said, "and I think he thought my feelings for him had, well, just sort of cooled off. It wasn't him. My feelings for everything had cooled off."

Margaret had been seeing a psychotherapist, who she hoped would help her overcome her depression and the anxiety she had been experiencing recently. At his suggestion, she was attending group therapy meetings. Also at his suggestion, she had gone to her physician to get a prescription for Zoloft (generic name *sertraline*), a serotonin-selective reuptake inhibitor. During the seven months Margaret had been taking Zoloft, her physician had increased her dosage twice after she had told him she wasn't feeling significantly better emotionally. "And physically, I'm not getting any better," she said. "If anything, I'm getting worse. I asked my doctor if I could be allergic to Zoloft, because I've really noticed that I feel worse, at least physically, since I started taking it. He just kind of smiled and patted my hand and said, 'Hang in there. These things take time.'"

"There's one other thing," she said. "I don't know if this means anything, but in the past couple of years, it's gotten so I'm incredibly sensitive to smells. I can hardly stand to go into a public building because the smell of perfume just makes me almost sick to my stomach. I practically have to cover my nose and run away. Jeff even had to stop wearing aftershave lotion. And cigarette smoke, don't even mention cigarette smoke. It seems like it's connected to the panicky feelings I have."

Although she was correct in her assessment that she didn't have a problem with recreational drugs, Margaret did have a drug problem. A *prescription* drug problem. In addition, in talking about being unnaturally sensitive to smells, she had described one the symptoms of multiple chemical sensitivities. Both her symptoms of anxiety and depression and her chemical sensitivities pointed to a problem associated with her body's inability to detoxify itself.

Her drug problem centered on the gradual dosage increases her physician had recommended. As Margaret's brain compensated for Zoloft's disruption of the serotonin production, release, and reuptake cycle, her symptoms would return. Her physician responded in a manner that has become all too typical: by prescribing higher doses of the drug to help her achieve "relief" from her symptoms. And in fact, although she was not, in the classic sense, *allergic* to Zoloft, the drug contributed significantly to a toxic load that was already overwhelming Margaret's ability to detoxify. By doing this, Zoloft almost certainly did make her feel physically worse.

The results of her Detoxification Profile, one of the diagnostic tests I ordered for Margaret, confirmed that her body's ability to detoxify was severely impaired. In addition, the tests pinpointed the problem: a breakdown in one of the stages of the detoxification process in the liver. Under normal circumstances, most toxins which have managed to enter the bloodstream pass through the liver, where they undergo a two-stage detoxification process. In Phase I detoxification, toxin molecules are oxidized by a family of enzymes, with each individual enzyme capable of acting on a number of different toxins. Phase I detoxification actually turns toxins into *free radicals*, molecules which are highly reactive with other molecular substances. Although free radicals can be very damaging elsewhere in the body, in the controlled environment of the liver, the free radical stage is required to prepare toxins for the next step in detoxification.

In Phase II detoxification, free radical toxin molecules are "conjugated." This means that the free radical combines with one of four types of molecule—glycine, glutathione, glucuronide, or sulfur—in the liver. Conjugated toxin molecules are then eliminated in one of two ways. Some are filtered by the kidneys and then pass out of the body in the urine, while others are excreted by the liver into the large intestine, from where they pass out of the body in the stool.

Margaret's initial-visit medical history and her slight response to Zoloft indicated that she was serotonin-deficient, and she had begun taking the Quick-Start nutrients which I prescribed to correct that condition. She also began taking the Power Recovery Program Detoxification nutrients. These would prove to be critical to her successful recovery, given her body's difficulty in getting rid of toxins. The most important of the nutrients in Margaret's treatment would be the sulfur nutrients—MSM, alpha lipoic acid, and glutathione—which support Phase I detoxification in the liver. Glycine, which along with glutathione supports Phase II liver detoxification, would also be important for her. In addition, I had her take as much vitamin C as she could tolerate without its causing diarrhea, and she regularly took 10,000 mg per day. This would help her system manage the high levels of free radicals elsewhere in her body while the ability of her liver to carry out Phase II detoxification was being restored. I also arranged for Margaret to gradually taper her use of Zoloft under supervised outpatient conditions over a two-month period.

Within four months, Margaret was virtually symptom-free. She had "mostly good days," she said. "The key is that my moods have stabilized," she went on. "I'm not *up* all the time, but I feel *right*. I don't have those terrible valleys that used to last for days. And no more Zoloft! You can't imagine what a relief it is not to live under this constant cloud, thinking, 'My God, am I going to have to take this stuff for the rest of my life?' I may not be well yet, but well is where I'm headed."

CONCLUSION

The three case histories in this chapter deal with what we're coming to understand may well be a problem, not only for substance abusers, but also for people suffering from many other often debilitating conditions, from mood disorders to chronic pain and fatigue. It may well be that many of the people who tend to abuse psychotropic substances are in fact self-medicating in an attempt to deal with symptoms of high toxic load. As we become more and more aware of just how toxic our environment and our food supply are, it's increasingly up to us to monitor our biochemical health through biochemical testing, and, where necessary, to take the steps such as those outlined here to deal with this problem in a natural, healthy, and effective way.

Conclusion

I want to take a final look back over some of the important ground we've covered, and I want to look ahead to what you can expect in your substance-free future. Among the things I'll talk about are the prevalence of nutritional deficiencies of many types that are so common today, and how we can use nutrition and support groups to help control some of the important factors in our lives, including stress and genetics, that often contribute to our need to use psychotropic substances.

BEYOND QUICK-START AND DETOXIFICATION: OTHER COMMON NUTRITIONAL DEFICIENCIES

As you were reading through the case histories in Parts Three and Four of this book, several things may have jumped out at you. I'm referring to deficiencies of specific nutrients which are common to almost all of the patients whose treatments I've presented here.

You may have noticed, for instance, that almost every one of the patients featured in the case histories has either a deficiency of Omega 3 essential fatty acids or symptoms that indicate a deficiency of this EFA. I can't emphasize too strongly the need for Omega 3 essential fatty acids in rebuilding cells, especially neurons, which have been damaged by substance use. Another thing that you may have picked up is that virtually all substance abusers are magnesium-deficient. (By the way, deficiencies of Omega 3 fatty acids and of magnesium are not limited to substance users. It's a safe bet that as many as 75 percent of all Americans are deficient in one or both of these important life-supporting nutrients.) Although the Quick-Start mineral supplements contain magnesium, I often find that treating severe magnesium deficiencies with higher doses of this nutrient is required to reverse this condition.

You might also have noticed that I prescribed phosphatidyl serine for several of the patients whose stories I've recounted. This nutrient is quite expensive, and I normally recommend it in cases of long-term substance use where a great deal of cell "rebuilding" is required. But, along with lecithin, phosphatidyl serine is extremely important in rebuilding damaged neurons and in correcting other cellular damage. Taking this nutrient will insure that you have one of the important tools for repairing the damage your substance use may have caused.

The Quick-Start nutrients provide a protocol which targets specific neurotransmitter shortages while, at the same time, giving a general program designed to correct a broad range of nutritional deficiencies. The Detoxification nutrients provide a general regimen for removing toxins and shoring up the body's ability to detoxify itself. The nutrients I've mentioned in this section are ones that can help alleviate some of the other chronic conditions that often accompany chronic substance abuse.

DEALING WITH STRESS

Your Quick-Start questionnaire answers can provide you with an excellent starting point for dealing with stress in your life by identifying your key neurotransmitter deficiencies. Stress depletes neurotransmitters, but it does not necessarily deplete the same neurotransmitters in everyone. Some people rapidly deplete their supplies of catecholamines when they're under stress, while others tend to deplete serotonin or GABA in stressful situations. By helping you identify your primary neurotransmitter deficiency or deficiencies, the Quick-Start questionnaires are most likely giving you a clue as to which neurotransmitters you deplete when you're under stress of any kind. Your answers are, in effect, saying, "If you're under a great deal of stress, make sure you take nutrients which will enable you to maintain the necessary levels of your primary neurotransmitters."

Everyone has "stress triggers." You'll often hear them referred to as "buttons" that can be pushed, and you'll hear people talk about having their "chains yanked." Whatever your "stress triggers," the first step is learning to recognize them before you resort to using drugs. Stress comes in a wide variety of forms, from the stress related to work to that associated with relationships. I've also talked about various kinds of biochemical stress, including, especially, immune system stress caused by excess toxic load and allergies.

Since emotional stress often triggers substance use, you should avoid or eliminate stress wherever you can, especially in the early stages of detoxification. For most people, however, this is simply not possible. If this is the case with you, the next best thing is to make sure you "gear up" your body so that it is better able to cope with the stress you do experience. Learn to recognize your personal stress signals. They're the way your body tells you it needs more than you're giving it to cope successfully with specific situations. Become familiar with your stress-fighting needs. If you tend to reach for high-carbohydrate foods when you're under stress, your body may be telling you it's having trouble producing enough serotonin. Or if you have difficulty getting motivated to do certain tasks or following tasks through to completion, you may be underproducing dopamine.

No matter what the source of the stress you experience, you need to keep your levels of "stress hormones" at their peak. As you've discovered, the best way to do that is to make sure that your body has the nutritional tools it needs to help you cope with stressful situations. In addition, managing stress in more conventional ways—such as through physical exercise, psychotherapy, or attending support groups such as AA—is important. By relieving the stress of physical inactivity, unfinished emotional "business," and isolation, these methods can actually help you maintain your biochemical balance by preserving the neurotransmitters that stress depletes.

OVERCOMING GENETIC PROBLEMS

The rapid advances of genetic science are making it clear that there is very likely some possibility of genetic susceptibility to virtually all psychotropic substance abuse, from nicotine to alcohol to stimulants to opiates. But in the final analysis, talking about genetic susceptibility to certain substances is just another way of saying that no two people are alike. As I've explained, the main component in genetic susceptibility is higher requirements for certain nutrients, and the Power Recovery Program can give you the means to counteract your genetic susceptibilities by identifying and correcting the nutritional deficiencies that your genetic makeup may have led to.

People with genetic susceptibilities to certain substances often find that biochemical testing is very useful in helping to pinpoint the biochemical imbalances that are unique to them. For instance, you may need twice as much selenium in your diet as someone else, simply because of genetic differences. Or you may need significantly more tyrosine than someone else simply because your brain is genetically less efficient than that other person's brain at processing tyrosine into dopamine. Biochemical testing can identify these genetic problem areas so that they can be overcome with nutritional supplementation. The same principle holds true for detoxification. Testing can identify problems you may have in detoxifying your body, problems which can be overcome by targeted nutritional supplementation.

The Power Recovery Program gives you the means to discover your unique biochemical profile, and to use this information to shore up deficiencies and eliminate toxicities which may have a genetic basis. If you know that you're genetically susceptible to alcohol abuse, for instance, use nutrients to compensate for your body's unique biochemical condition. You may find that keeping your substance use under control is more of a challenge than it would be for someone without a high genetic vulnerability, but always remember that you can make up for genetics with nutrients.

THE IMPORTANCE OF NUTRITION TO DEVELOPING BRAINS

It is, of course, clear by now that I place the highest emphasis on providing the nutrients necessary to children and young adults so that their brains can develop fully. Of the utmost importance to ensuring that they are able to develop intellectually and emotionally is the avoidance of psychotropic substances. As I've pointed out, alcohol and drugs, both prescription and recreational, achieve their effects by disrupting neurotransmitters, especially in the frontal lobes of our brains. Neuroimagery (brain scans) show that this area of the brain is critical to the processes, including decision-making, empathy, and the ability to understand the consequences of behaviors, which define us as human. Psychotropic substances not only disrupt and delay the development of the frontal lobes in young people, but they also may actually prevent the full development from taking place at all.

I've also noted that the frontal lobes are the last areas of the brain to fully mature. For this reason, it is imperative that children and young adults be given the proper nutrition—especially the essential fatty acids and the amino acids, vitamins, and minerals that support proper neurotransmitter function—to enable them to develop fully as human beings. There is no better reason that I can think of to provide children with proper nutrition and a drug-free environment. It's one of the most important things we can do to secure their futures.

A PLACE FOR THERAPY AND SUPPORT GROUPS

The Power Recovery Program concentrates heavily on the biochemical aspect of overcoming substance problems by emphasizing the use of nutritional supplements to rebalance your biochemistry and detoxify your body. While it's not the place of this book to focus on the emotional and psychological problems that are often present in the lives of substance abusers, I would like to briefly discuss them here. There is no question that emotional stress can play a critical part in contributing to biochemical imbalances. It's also a fact that, for many people, recovering from substance problems necessarily involves confronting emotional or psychological problems, often with the help of a therapist. But I want to point out one other thing that is absolutely critical to understanding why the Power Recovery Program has proven so successful: It is, in most cases, pointless to spend extensive time in counseling or therapy to try to resolve emotional issues if you have not first at least begun the process of rebalancing your biochemistry.

For most of my patients, rebalancing their biochemistry and reestablishing normal brain chemistry has been the secret to overcoming mental and emotional disorders. Although I've heard it thousands of times, it still literally gives me chills of joy when I hear patients tell me that their emotional problems have become so much less significant in their lives. Let me give you some examples of how they express it:

"You know, since I've been taking the nutrients you prescribed, I'm a warmer, friendlier person. I'm not angry all the time."

"I can *think* again. I didn't realize how brain-fogged I'd been. I can see my way through problems that used to just make me angry or frustrated because I couldn't figure out how to deal with them."

"I still go to AA meetings, and AA has been very important in my life. But, you know what-don't get me wrong, but I think I've moved past the AA stage. It was necessary, but it's not any longer. And I know AA will always be there for me for tough issues."

"My problems didn't go away, but they sure did change a hell of a lot. When I look back at some of the things I used to get upset about, I can't believe it. I can literally deal with life now. And I don't need drugs to do it. In fact, drugs were actually preventing me from dealing with it, not helping me."

Don't misunderstand. I appreciate and support the role that psychological and pastoral counseling, spirituality, and support groups can play in helping people sort out difficult problems. But based on the testimony of so many of my patients, I can tell you that as you restore biochemical balance to your life, you're taking the single most important step toward restoring psychological and emotional balance as well. The idea that there needs to be a psychotropic drug to help us through any crisis we might face is one of the most dangerous and dehumanizing, as well as widespread, tenets held by those in medical practice today. The Power Recovery Program gives you the means to demonstrate just how wrong that idea is. By rebalancing your brain chemistry, you'll be providing yourself with a critical resource to realize the full benefits of counseling and support groups and to fully understand, cope with, and overcome even the most difficult emotional and psychological problems in your life.

A FINAL WORD

If you've successfully completed the Quick-Start stage and are well into Detoxification, you've probably got a good idea of what "makes you tick," of what specific neurotransmitters are key for you. And if you've taken your recovery a step further and have had some biochemical tests done, you've got an even better idea of what you need in order to feel good, think clearly, and function well without drugs or alcohol. Whatever your biochemical profile, use your knowledge of it to keep yourself in top emotional and intellectual form by continuing to take your personal program of nutritional supplements. Because that's what the Power Recovery Program is really all about: helping you design a personal protocol of nutritional supplementation that will enable you to fully realize the physical, emotional, and intellectual joys of living healthy and substance-free.

In Chapter 2, I talked about the fact that technology has enabled us to "supercharge" psychotropic substances, making them much more powerful and more addictive than their natural counterparts. But the converse of that is also true. Technology has enabled us to isolate, concentrate, and deliver *nutrients* in ways that were unimaginable half of a century ago. We are now able to identify nutritional deficiencies and correct them by using the specific nutrient substances, including amino acids, vitamins and phytonutrients, minerals, fats, and enzymes, that technology enables us to isolate. It's one way in which we can fight technology with technology.

One of the most important things this has enabled us to do is to fully realize the miracle of our billion-year-old biochemistry. We have the opportunity today, as never before in history, to understand and bring ourselves into harmony with this ancient biochemistry. In doing so, we also bring ourselves closer spiritually to being able to fulfill our destinies in life.

I like happy endings. Perhaps I should rephrase that: I like happy new beginnings. You've no doubt noticed that the case histories I've presented all end on a positive note. This does not mean that some of my patients aren't able to overcome their problems. I wish I could report a 100 percent success rate, but, of course, I can't. The Power Recovery Program has, however, achieved the highest success rates of any clinically documented program. I feel justified in emphasizing the positive because so many of my patients *do* get well. The happy endings you've read about are not fiction, and they're the rule rather than the exception. And as you use the Power Recovery Program to overcome your substance problem, I have no doubt you'll be writing your own happy ending. Or should I say, your own happy new beginning.

APPENDIX A

Nutritional Supplement Checklists

In this section, I've included checklists of the nutritional supplements for each of the five Quick-Start programs and for Detoxification. There is a box for morning, afternoon, and evening doses for each day of the week. Each checklist will enable you to track one week's worth of supplements. Many of my patients find that having checklists such as the ones I include here is very effective in helping them keep track of their recovery. Many also keep notes on their checklists as to how they feel at different stages of their recovery.

Before you start, you might want to photocopy the checklist for your Quick-Start program(s) and for Detoxification so you can use them to track several weeks' worth of supplements. Using the checklists will help you monitor your supplement usage accurately.

If you're a smoker, notice that I've included cigarette counters as well. Check off your cigarette counter each time you smoke a cigarette. This way you'll be able to track the reduction in your cigarette consumption as you go through the Quick-Start for Smokers program.

Below are weekly charts which can be used to track your supplementation.

CATECHOLAMINE DEFICIENCY NUTRITIONAL SUPPLEMENT **CHECKLIST**

Supplements	Dosage	Day 1			Day 2		
B Vitamin Capsule	1/3 of daily dosage	AM	PM	EVE	AM	PM	EVE
Multimineral	1/3 of daily dosage	AM	PM	EVE	AM	PM	EVE
L-Glutamine	Up to 1,000 mg	AM	PM	EVE	AM	PM	EVE
L-Tyrosine	Up to 1,500 mg	AM	PM	EVE	AM	PM	EVE
Vitamin C	Up to 500 mg	AM	PM	EVE	AM	PM	EVE

SEROTONIN DEFICIENCY NUTRITIONAL SUPPLEMENT **CHECKLIST**

Supplements	Dosage	Day 1			Day 2		
B Vitamin Capsule	1/3 of daily dosage	AM	PM	EVE	AM	PM	EVE
Multimineral	1/3 of daily dosage	AM	PM	EVE	AM	PM	EVE
L-Glutamine	Up to 1,000 mg	AM	PM	EVE	AM	PM	EVE
5HTP	Up to 300 mg	AM	PM	EVE	AM	PM	EVE

Please duplicate for your personal needs.

WEEK # _____

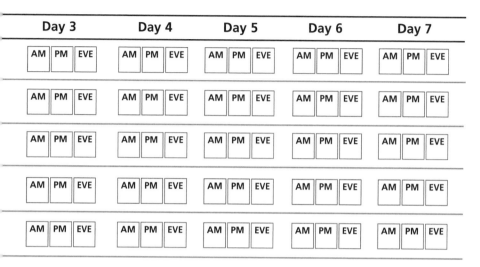

WEEK # _____

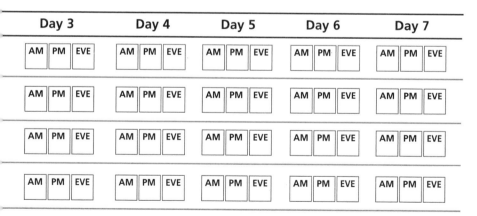

Below are weekly charts which can be used to track your supplementation.

GABA DEFICIENCY NUTRITIONAL SUPPLEMENT **CHECKLIST**

Supplements	Dosage	Day 1	Day 2
B Vitamin Capsule	1/3 of daily dosage	AM PM EVE	AM PM EVE
Multimineral	1/3 of daily dosage	AM PM EVE	AM PM EVE
L-Glutamine	Up to 3,500 mg	AM PM EVE	AM PM EVE
L-Taurine	Up to 1,000 mg	AM PM EVE	AM PM EVE

ENDORPHIN/ENKEPHALIN DEFICIENCY NUTRITIONAL SUPPLEMENT **CHECKLIST**

Supplements	Dosage	Day 1	Day 2
B Vitamin Capsule	1/3 of daily dosage	AM PM EVE	AM PM EVE
Multimineral	1/3 of daily dosage	AM PM EVE	AM PM EVE
L-Glutamine	Up to 1,000 mg	AM PM EVE	AM PM EVE
DL-Phenylalanine	Up to 2,000 mg	AM PM EVE	AM PM EVE
L-Leucine	Up to 500 mg	AM PM EVE	AM PM EVE
L-Methionine	Up to 500 mg	AM PM EVE	AM PM EVE

Please duplicate for your personal needs.

WEEK # _____

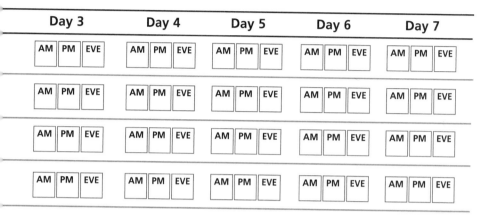

WEEK # _____

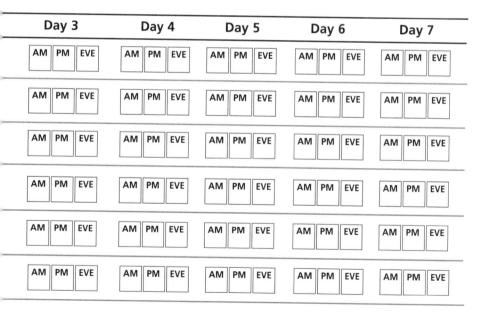

Below is a weekly chart which can be used to track your supplementation.

QUICK-START FOR SMOKERS NUTRITIONAL SUPPLEMENT **CHECKLIST**

Supplements	Dosage	Day 1			Day 2		
B Vitamin Capsule	1/3 of daily dosage	AM	PM	EVE	AM	PM	EVE
Multimineral	1/3 of daily dosage	AM	PM	EVE	AM	PM	EVE
L-Glutamine	Up to 1,000 mg	AM	PM	EVE	AM	PM	EVE
L-Tyrosine	Up to 1,000 mg	AM	PM	EVE	AM	PM	EVE
5HTP	Up to 100 mg	AM	PM	EVE	AM	PM	EVE
Phosphatidyl Choline	Up to 1,000 mg	AM	PM	EVE	AM	PM	EVE

Cigarette Counter (Day 1) 1 2 3 4 5 6 7 8 9 10 11 12 13 14 15 16 17 18 19

Cigarette Counter (Day 2) 1 2 3 4 5 6 7 8 9 10 11 12 13 14 15 16 17 18 19

Cigarette Counter (Day 3) 1 2 3 4 5 6 7 8 9 10 11 12 13 14 15 16 17 18 19

Cigarette Counter (Day 4) 1 2 3 4 5 6 7 8 9 10 11 12 13 14 15 16 17 18 19

Cigarette Counter (Day 5) 1 2 3 4 5 6 7 8 9 10 11 12 13 14 15 16 17 18 19

Cigarette Counter (Day 6) 1 2 3 4 5 6 7 8 9 10 11 12 13 14 15 16 17 18 19

Cigarette Counter (Day 7) 1 2 3 4 5 6 7 8 9 10 11 12 13 14 15 16 17 18 19

Please duplicate for your personal needs.

WEEK # _____

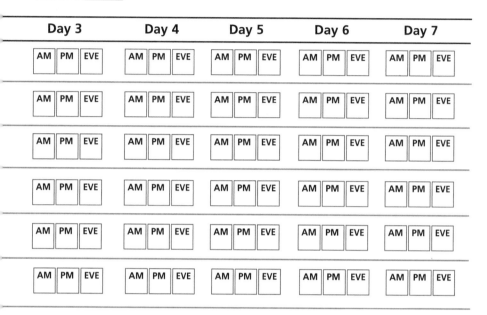

Day 3	Day 4	Day 5	Day 6	Day 7
AM PM EVE	AM PM EVE	AM PM EVE	AM PM EVE	AM PM EVE
AM PM EVE	AM PM EVE	AM PM EVE	AM PM EVE	AM PM EVE
AM PM EVE	AM PM EVE	AM PM EVE	AM PM EVE	AM PM EVE
AM PM EVE	AM PM EVE	AM PM EVE	AM PM EVE	AM PM EVE
AM PM EVE	AM PM EVE	AM PM EVE	AM PM EVE	AM PM EVE
AM PM EVE	AM PM EVE	AM PM EVE	AM PM EVE	AM PM EVE

20 21 22 23 24 25 26 27 28 29 30 31 32 33 34 35 36 37 38 39 40

20 21 22 23 24 25 26 27 28 29 30 31 32 33 34 35 36 37 38 39 40

20 21 22 23 24 25 26 27 28 29 30 31 32 33 34 35 36 37 38 39 40

20 21 22 23 24 25 26 27 28 29 30 31 32 33 34 35 36 37 38 39 40

20 21 22 23 24 25 26 27 28 29 30 31 32 33 34 35 36 37 38 39 40

20 21 22 23 24 25 26 27 28 29 30 31 32 33 34 35 36 37 38 39 40

20 21 22 23 24 25 26 27 28 29 30 31 32 33 34 35 36 37 38 39 40

Below is a weekly chart which can be used to track your supplementation.

DETOXIFICATION NUTRITIONAL SUPPLEMENT **CHECKLIST**

Supplements	Dosage	Day 1		Day 2	
Phosphatidyl Choline	Up to 2,000 mg	AM	PM	AM	PM
Lactobacillus	2.5 billion org.	AM	PM	AM	PM
Bifidus	2.5 billion org.	AM	PM	AM	PM
Vitamin E	Up to 400 IU	AM	PM	AM	PM
Vitamin C	Up to 2,500 mg	AM	PM	AM	PM
MSM	Up to 2,000 mg	AM	PM	AM	PM
Alpha Lipoic Acid	Up to 300 mg	AM	PM	AM	PM
Glutathione	Up to 100 mg	AM	PM	AM	PM
Glycine	Up to 1,500 mg	AM	PM	AM	PM

Please duplicate for your personal needs.

WEEK # _____

Day 3	Day 4	Day 5	Day 6	Day 7
AM PM	AM PM	AM PM	AM PM	AM PM
AM PM	AM PM	AM PM	AM PM	AM PM
AM PM	AM PM	AM PM	AM PM	AM PM
AM PM	AM PM	AM PM	AM PM	AM PM
AM PM	AM PM	AM PM	AM PM	AM PM
AM PM	AM PM	AM PM	AM PM	AM PM
AM PM	AM PM	AM PM	AM PM	AM PM
AM PM	AM PM	AM PM	AM PM	AM PM
AM PM	AM PM	AM PM	AM PM	AM PM

Resources for Purchasing Nutritional Supplements and Supporting Recovery

Many of my patients ask for recommendations when it comes to buying nutritional supplements and seeking additional support. Thankfully, I can safely refer you to the following companies, organizations, and centers. I am very familiar with all of the facilities recommended below, and I trust their integrity

SOURCES OF QUALITY NUTRITIONAL SUPPLEMENTS

One of the most important recommendations I can make is that you purchase only the purest, highest-quality nutritional supplements for use in your Power Recovery Program. Unfortunately, that means that I simply cannot recommend over-the-counter supplements, with a few exceptions. Here are three sources for purchasing nutritional supplements that I highly recommend:

Nutrenergy Pathways
1-800-614-7714
www.NuPathways.com
"NuPathways" sells the highest quality nutritional supplements in packs specially configured for the Power Recovery Program. Through NuPathways you can purchase Quick-Start nutritional supplement packs specifically designed to help you recover from each of the four neurotransmitter deficiencies and for smokers and marijuana users.

Nutritional Therapeutics Inc. (NTI)
1-800-982-9158

NTI is a source of high-quality, pure, and extremely absorbable nutrients. Products can be ordered by phone or purchased in many health food stores.

Thorne Nutraceuticals
1-800-228-1966

Thorne is an excellent source of high-quality nutrients. Products can be ordered by phone or purchased in many health food stores.

SUPPORT ORGANIZATIONS AND FACILITIES

Below you will find organizations and facilities that can provide you with further information, practical assistance, and support. If you wish to contact Dr. Gant to learn more about his unique approach to substance use problems, you can do so through either Connected Pathways LLC or National Integrated Health Associates (NIHA).

Alliance for Addictions Solutions (AAS)
www.AllianceForAddictionsSolutions.org

AAS is an organization of treatment providers, people in recovery, and concerned citizens. Those affiliated with this organization support nutritional and integrative medicine healing approaches and other non-pharmacological interventions for treating addictions.

Alternative to Meds Center
1-800-359-9698
www.alternativetomedscenter.com

This rehabilitation facility is located in San Francisco, CA. It uses nutrition-based approaches to substance abuse rehabilitation that are compatible with the Power Recover Program.

Bridging the Gaps
1-866-711-1234
www.bridgingthegaps.com

This rehabilitation facility is located in Winchester, VA. It uses nutrition-based approaches to substance abuse rehabilitation that are compatible with the Power Recover Program.

Connected Pathways LLC
1-888-847-4233

www.connectedpathways.com

Connected Pathways provides counseling and community support for people in recovery who are following the Power Recovery Program as outlined in this book. Connected Pathways also provides customized nutritional supplement formulations based on biochemical testing results as outlined in the Long-Term Biochemical Rebalancing section of this book. And Connected Pathways provides instruction for clinicians who wish to use the Power Recovery Program with their clients.

G&G Holistic Addiction Treatment Program
1-800-559-9503

www.holisticdrugrehab.com

This rehabilitation facility is located in Miami, FL. It uses nutrition-based approaches to substance abuse rehabilitation that are compatible with the Power Recover Program.

National Integrated Health Associates (NIHA)
1-202-237-7000

www.nihadc.com

NIHA is a leading holistic and integrative medical and dental practice serving the Washington, DC, Maryland, and Northern Virginia metropolitan area. NIHA's professional health team is comprised of holistic medical doctors, biological dentists, naturopaths, and other health professionals. Merging traditional medicine with complementary and alternative medicine (CAM), the staff supports and empowers patients along their journey to health and wellness.

Weston A. Price Foundation
www.WestonAPrice.org

The Weston A. Price Foundation is one of the best resources for dietary information that I've found. You'll find information on how to follow the best possible diet for supporting your recovery through eating clean, nutrient-dense foods.

Bibliography

The following sources provide background for many of the basic topics covered in this book, including the effects of nutrients on brain function, the role of nutritional and biochemical imbalances in the development of substance problems, and the use of nutritional therapy to treat substance problems. Thousands of books and articles are relevant to these topics, and the entries I've cited are not meant to be comprehensive. They will, however, provide you with a starting point on which you can base further research.

Beasley, Joseph D. *Diagnosing and Managing Chemical Dependency.* Amityville, NY: 1992.

Beasley, Joseph D. *Wrong Diagnosis, Wrong Treatment: The Plight of the Alcoholic in America.* New York, NY: 1987.

Beasley, Joseph D., and Jerry J. Swift. "Dietary Intake of Certain Amino Acids Linked to Brain Function," *Clinical Psychiatry,* 8:10 (1980), pp. 1–20.

Beasley, Joseph D., and Jerry J. Swift. *The Kellogg Report: The Impact of Nutrition, Environment, & Lifestyle on the Health of Americans.* Annandale-on-Hudson, NY: The Institute of Health Policy and Practice, Bard College Center, 1989.

Biederman, J., et al. "Family-Environmental Risk Factors for Attention Deficit Hyperactivity Disorder," *Archives of General Psychiatry,* Vol. 52, June 1995, pp. 464–470.

Blum, Kenneth. *Alcohol and the Addictive Brain.* New York, NY: The Free Press, 1991.

Breggin, Peter. *Toxic Psychiatry.* New York, NY: St. Martin's Press, 1990.

Coppen, A., et al. "Tryptophan Metabolism in Depressive Illness," *Psychological Medicine,* Vol. 4 (1974), pp. 164–173.

De Duve, Christian. *A Guided Tour of the Living Cell.* New York, NY: Scientific American Library, 1984.

Dipalma, Joseph. "Magnesium Replacement Therapy," *AFP Clinical Pharmacology,* July 1980.

Dressler, David, and Huntington Potter. *Discovering Enzymes.* New York, NY: Scientific American Library, 1991.

Fox, A. "Phenylalanine: Resistance to Disease Through Nutrition," *Let's Live,* November 1983, pp. 16–26.

Gant, Charles E. *Alternative and Bionutritional Approaches to ADD and ADHD.* Syracuse, NY: AFCO, 1997.

Geidenberg, A., et al. "Tyrosine for the Treatment of Depression," *American Journal of Psychiatry,* 1984, 137:622–632.

Gelenberg, A. J., and R.J. Wurtman. "Tyrosine for Depression," *Lancet,* October 1980.

Goodsell, David S. *The Machinery of Life.* New York, NY: Springer-Verlag, 1993.

Growden, J.H., et al. "Treatment of Brain Diseases with Dietary Precursors of Neurotransmitters," *Annals of Internal Medicine,* 80:10 (1980), pp. 1638–1639.

Guenther, R.M. "Role of Nutritional Therapy in Alcoholism Treatment," *International Journal of Biosocial Research*, 4:1 (1983), pp. 5–18.

Haddad, L.M. "Managing Tricyclic Antidepressant Overdose," *American Family Physician*, 46 (1) July 1992, pp. 153–159.

Hendler, Nelson. "Depression Caused by Chronic Pain," *Journal of Clinical Psychiatry*, 45:3 (1984), pp. 30–36.

Hunnisett, A. "Gut Fermentation (or the 'Auto-Brewery') Syndrome," *Journal of Nutritional Medicine*, Vol. 1, 1990, pp. 33–38.

Kukreja, R.C., and M.L. Hess. *Free Radicals, Cardiovascular Dysfunction and Protection Strategies*. Austin, CO: R.G. Landes Company, 1994.

Larson, Joan Mathews. *Seven Weeks to Sobriety*. New York, NY: Fawcett Columbine, 1997.

Leutwyler, K. "Paying Attention: The Controversy Over ADHD and the Drug Ritalin is Obscuring a Real Look at the Disorder and Its Underpinnings," *Scientific American*, August 1996, pp. 12–13.

Lieber, Charles S. *Medical and Nutritional Complications of Alcoholism*. New York and London: Plenum Medical Book Company, 1994.

Maher, T.J. "Tyrosine, Catecholamines, and Brain Function," *The Nutrition Report*, Vol. 3, No. 6, June 1990.

Nahas, G.G., and C. Latour, eds. *Cannabis: Physiopathology, Epidemiology, Detection*. Boca Raton, FL: CRC Press, 1993.

Pomerleau, O.F., et al. "Neuroendocrine Reactivity to Nicotine in Smokers," *Psychopharmacology*, Vol. 81, 1983, pp. 61–67.

Poser, W., et al. "Mortality in Patients with Dependence on Prescription Drugs," *Drug-Alcohol Dependence*, 30 (1), April 1992, pp. 49–57.

Reinstein, D.K., H. Lehnert, and R.J. Wurtman. "Neurochemical and Behavioral Consequences of Stress: Effects of Dietary Tyrosine," *Journal of the American College of Nutrition*, 3 (3), 1984.

Schuckit, M. "Alcoholic Patients with Secondary Depression," *American Journal of Psychiatry*, 14:6 (1983), pp. 711–714.

Shabert, Judy, and Nancy Ehrlich. *The Ultimate Nutrient: Glutamine*. Garden City Park, NY: Avery Publishing Group, 1994.

Simonson, Melvin. "L-Phenylalanine," *Journal of Clinical Psychiatry*, 46:8 (1985), p. 355.

Slagle, Priscilla. *The Way Up From Down*. New York, NY: Random House, 1992.

Stevens, L. "Essential Fatty Acid Metabolism in Boys With ADHD," *American Journal of Clinical Nutrition*, 1995, 62:761–768.

Ticku, M. "Alcohol and GABA-Benzodiazepine Receptor Function," *Annals of Medicine*, Vol. 22, 1990, pp. 241–246.

Vereby, K., ed. *Opioids in Mental Illness: Theories, Clinical Observations, and Treatment Possibilities*. Annals of the New York Academy of Sciences, Vol. 398, 1982, pp. 487–497.

Volkow, N.D. "Is Methylphenidate (Ritalin) Like Cocaine?" *Archives of General Psychiatry*, Vol. 52, June 1995, pp. 456–463.

Volkow, N.D., et al. "Dopamine Transporter Occupancies in the Human Brain Induced by Therapeutic Doses of Methylphenidate (Ritalin)," *American Journal of Psychiatry*, Vol. 155 (10), October 1998, pp. 1325–1331.

Walker, Sydney. *The Hyperactivity Hoax*. New York, NY: St. Martin's Press, 1998.

Werbach, Melvyn R. *Foundations of Nutritional Medicine: A Sourcebook of Clinical Research*. Tarzana, CA: Third Line Press, Inc., 1997.

Will, George. "The Doping of America's Kids," *New York Post*, December 2, 1999, p. 32.

Wood, D.R., et al. "Treatment of Attention Deficit Disorder With DL-Phenylalanine," *Psychiatry Resources*, Vol. 16, 1985, pp. 21–26.

Wurtman, R.J. "Nutrients That Modify Brain Function," *Scientific American*, Vol. 246 (1982), pp. 50–59.

Index

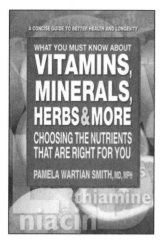

WHAT YOU MUST KNOW ABOUT VITAMINS, MINERALS, HERBS & MORE

Choosing the Nutrients That Are Right for You

Pamela Wartian Smith, MD, MPH

Almost 75 percent of your health and life expectancy is based on lifestyle, environment, and nutrition. Yet even if you follow a healthful diet, you are probably not getting all the nutrients you need to prevent disease. In *What You Must Know About Vitamins, Minerals, Herbs & More,* Dr. Pamela Smith explains how you can restore and maintain health through the wise use of nutrients.

Part One of this easy-to-use guide discusses the individual nutrients necessary for good health. Part Two offers personalized nutritional programs for people with a wide variety of health concerns. People without prior medical problems can look to Part Three for their supplementation plans. Whether you want to maintain good health or you are trying to overcome a medical condition, *What You Must Know About Vitamins, Minerals, Herbs & More,* can help you make the best choices for the health and well-being of you and your family.

$15.95 • 448 pages • 6 x 9-inch quality paperback • ISBN 978-0-7570-0233-5

DETOX AND REVITALIZE

The Holistic Guide for Renewing
Your Body, Mind, and Spirit

Susana L. Belen

Even if you try to follow a healthy diet and lifestyle, toxins and waste materials accumulate in your cells, compromising your health. But help is at hand. Part One of *Detox and Revitalize* explains the need for detoxification, and guides you in purifying your body. Part Two presents taste-tempting recipes for grains, cereals, and legumes; beverages; salads; soups; main dishes; and even sweets that will increase your vitality. Chapters on herbs and home remedies round out this easy-to-use guide.

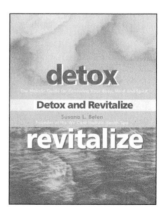

$14.95 • 160 pages • 8 x 10-inch quality paperback • ISBN 978-1-890612-46-7

THE SQUARE ONE HEALTH GUIDES

Written by health professionals who are well recognized in their respective fields, the following concise, easy-to-read books focus on a wide range of important health concerns. From migraine headaches to high cholesterol, each title looks at a specific problem; each provides a clear explanation of the disorder, its causes, and its symptoms; and each offers natural solutions that can either greatly reduce or completely eliminate the problem. Some titles also focus on natural alternatives to drugs with serious side effects—alternatives that in many cases can be used in conjunction with prescription medications. This growing series of titles can be counted on to provide safe and sensible solutions to all-too-common health problems.

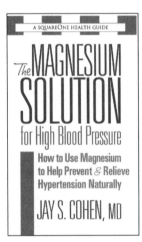

THE MAGNESIUM SOLUTION FOR HIGH BLOOD PRESSURE
How to Use Magnesium to Help Prevent & Relieve Hypertension Naturally

Jay S. Cohen, MD

Approximately 50 percent of Americans have hypertension. While many medications are available to combat this condition, they come with potential side effects. Fortunately, there is a remedy that's both safe and effective—magnesium. *The Magnesium Solution for High Blood Pressure* describes the best types of magnesium, explores appropriate dosage, and details the use of magnesium with hypertension meds.

$5.95 • 96 pages • 4 x 7-inch mass paperback • ISBN 978-0-7570-0255-7

THE MAGNESIUM SOLUTION FOR MIGRAINE HEADACHES
How to Use Magnesium to Prevent and Relieve Migraine & Cluster Headaches Naturally

Jay S. Cohen, MD

More than 30 million people in North America suffer from migraine headaches. While a number of drugs are used to treat migraines, they come with a risk of side effects. But there is a safe alternative—magnesium. This guide shows how magnesium can treat migraines, and pinpoints the best magnesium to use and the proper dosage.

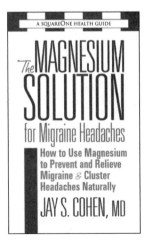

$5.95 • 96 pages • 4 x 7-inch mass paperback • ISBN 978-0-7570-0256-4